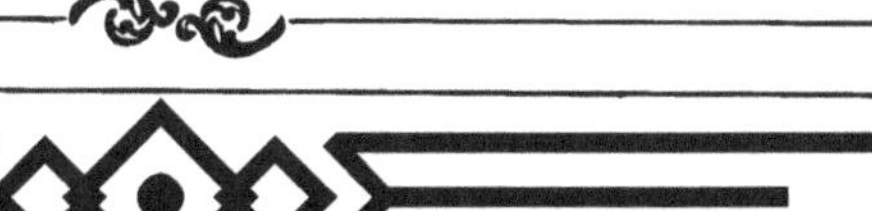

2024
Edition

LYMPHEDEMA DIET FOR BEGINNERS

Nourishing Recipes for Managing Lymphedema

with a 30-Day Healthy Eating Challenge

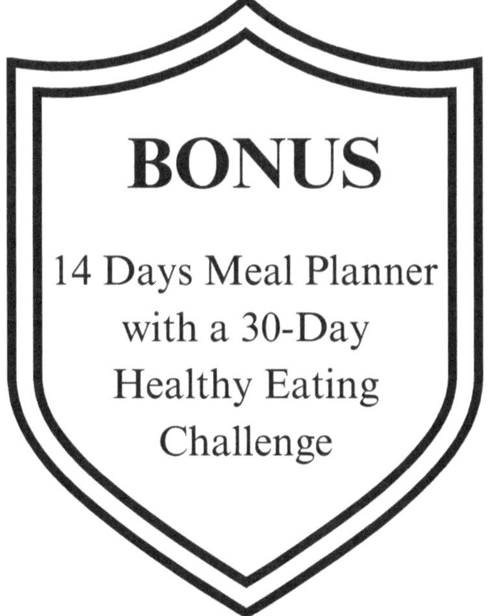

VAKARE RIMKUTE

Copyright © 2024 by Vakare Rimkute

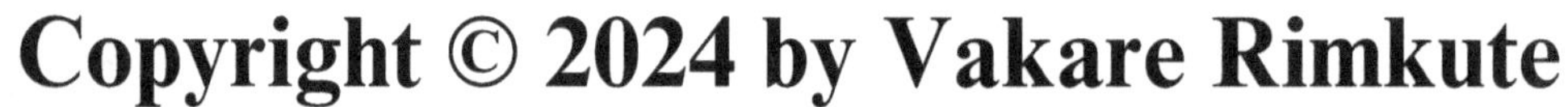 Disclaimer

The recipes and information presented in this cookbook are intended for general informational purposes only. While Vakare Rimkute has made every effort to ensure the accuracy and completeness of the content, they make no representations or warranties of any kind, express or implied, about the suitability or applicability of the recipes for any purpose .

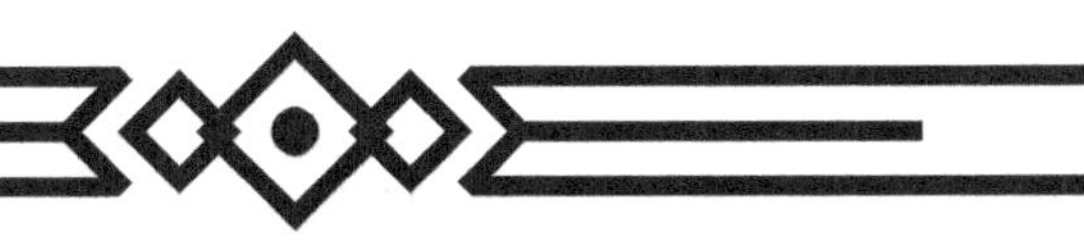

INTRODUCTION TO LYMPHEDEMA

Lymphedema, characterized by the swelling of tissues due to the accumulation of lymph fluid, has been recognized by medical practitioners for centuries. Ancient medical texts from civilizations such as ancient *Egypt* and Greece describe symptoms resembling those of lymphedema. However, it wasn't until the **19th and 20th centuries** that significant advancements in medical understanding and treatment began to emerge.

During the 19th century, physicians like **William and James Turner** published works shedding light on the lymphatic system's role in maintaining fluid balance within the body. However, effective treatments remained elusive, and lymphedema often led to debilitating complications for those affected.

The 20th century marked a turning point in the understanding and management of lymphedema. Pioneering surgeons such as **Dr. Emil Vodder** developed manual lymphatic drainage (MLD) techniques in the 1930s, laying the foundation for modern lymphedema therapy. Furthermore, the development of surgical procedures, such as lymphaticovenular anastomosis (LVA) and vascularized lymph node transfer (VLNT), in the latter half of the 20th century provided new hope for those with lymphedema.

Despite significant progress, lymphedema continues to present challenges for patients and healthcare providers alike. Factors such as limited access to specialized care, misconceptions about the condition, and inadequate support systems can hinder effective management. However, recent decades have also witnessed remarkable advancements in non-invasive treatments, such as compression therapy, exercise programs, and nutritional interventions.

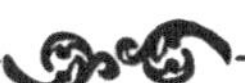

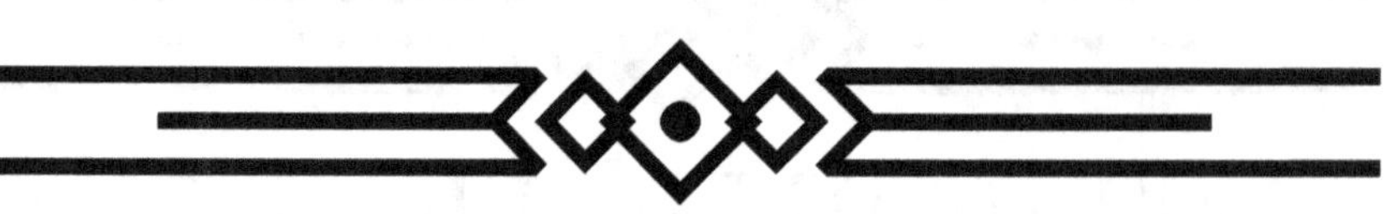

As our understanding of lymphedema deepens and technology advances, there is hope for even more effective treatments and improved quality of life for individuals living with this condition. This cookbook aims to complement existing therapeutic approaches by providing nutritious and delicious recipes tailored to support lymphedema management. Through a combination of culinary creativity and evidence-based nutrition, we strive to empower individuals to take control of their health and well-being.

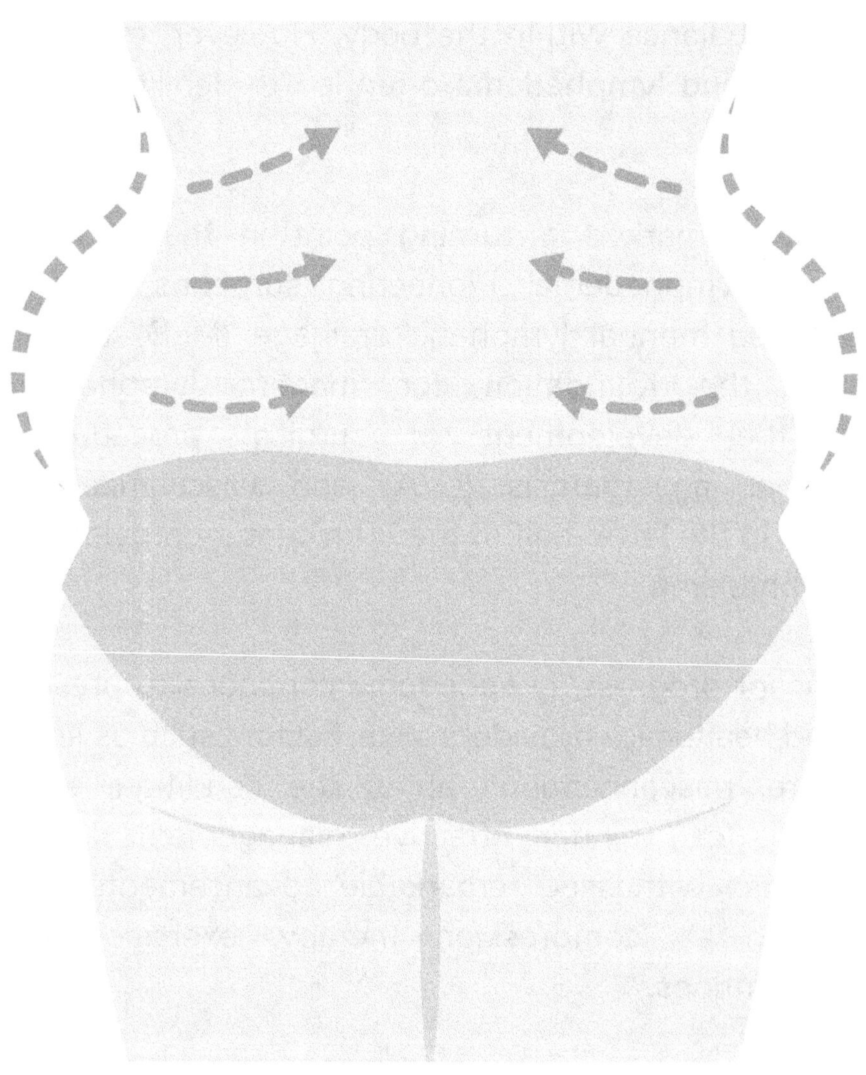

TABLE

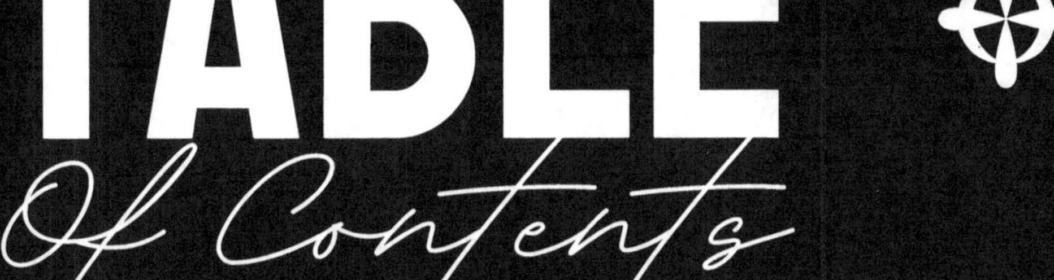

Of Contents

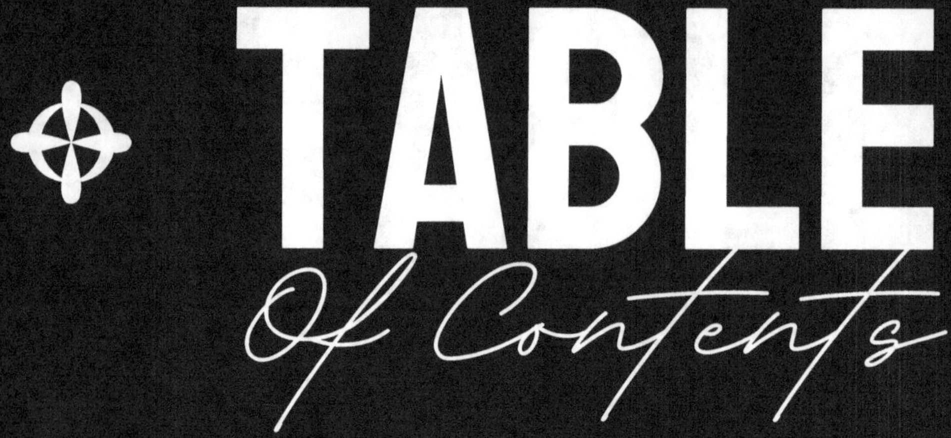
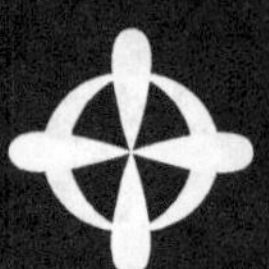

TABLE
Of Contents

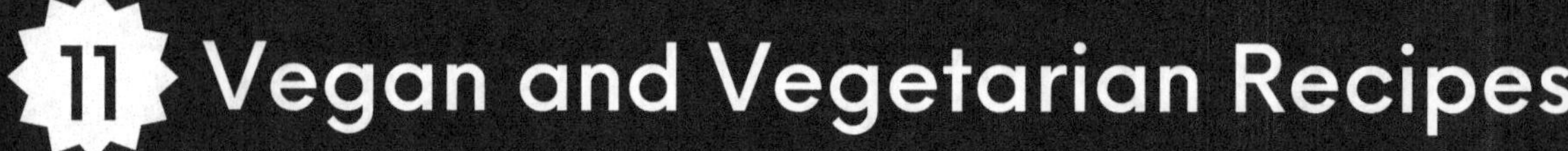

Chapter 1

Introduction to Lymphedema and Nutrition

WHAT IS LYMPHEDEMA

Lymphedema is a chronic condition characterized by the accumulation of lymph fluid in the body's tissues, leading to swelling, typically in the arms or legs. This swelling occurs when the lymphatic system, responsible for draining excess fluid from tissues and transporting immune cells throughout the body, is impaired or damaged.

There are two main types of lymphedema:

1. **Primary lymphedema**: This type occurs due to abnormalities in the development of the lymphatic system, often present at birth or manifesting later in life without an identifiable cause.

2. **Secondary lymphedema**: This type develops as a result of damage to the lymphatic system, commonly due to surgery (such as lymph node removal during cancer treatment), radiation therapy, infection, trauma, or other medical conditions.

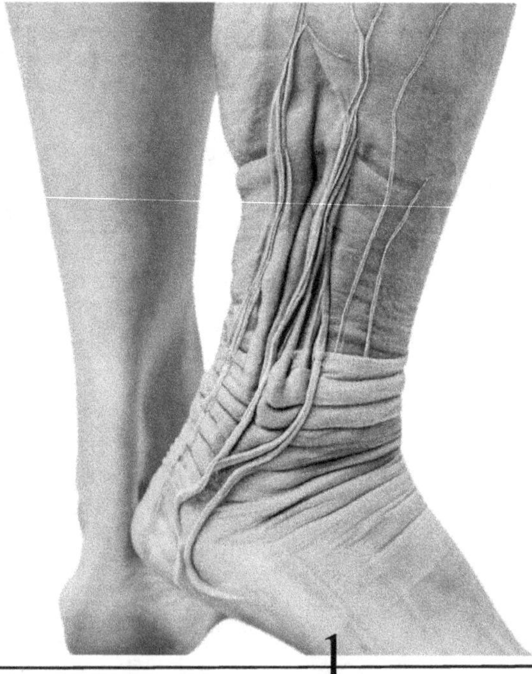

CAUSES OF LYMPHEDEMA

1. **Surgery**: Lymph node removal or damage during surgeries such as mastectomy (common in breast cancer treatment) can disrupt the lymphatic system's function, leading to lymphedema.
2. **Radiation Therapy:** Radiation treatment aimed at lymph nodes or surrounding tissues can cause scarring and damage to the lymphatic vessels, resulting in lymphedema.
3. **Cancer**: Lymphedema can occur as a result of cancer itself, particularly cancers that affect the lymphatic system, such as lymphoma. Additionally, tumours pressing on lymphatic vessels can impede fluid drainage.
4. **Infection**: Infections such as cellulitis can cause inflammation and damage to the lymphatic vessels, leading to impaired lymphatic drainage and subsequent swelling.
5. **Injury or Trauma**: Severe injury or trauma, including burns or trauma to the lymphatic system, can disrupt lymphatic flow and contribute to lymphedema.

SYMPTOMS OF LYMPHEDEMA

1. **Swelling**: Persistent swelling, often in one arm or leg, but can also affect other areas of the body.
2. **Feeling of Heaviness or Tightness**: The affected limb may feel heavy, tight, or full due to fluid buildup.
3. **Decreased Range of Motion**: Swelling and tissue changes can limit movement in the affected limb.
4. **Pain or Discomfort:** Some individuals may experience discomfort, aching, or even pain in the affected area.
5. **Recurrent Infections**: Due to compromised lymphatic function, individuals with lymphedema may be more susceptible to infections like cellulitis in the affected limb.

ROLE OF DIET IN LYMPHEDEMA MANAGEMENT

1. **Sodium Intake**: High sodium consumption can lead to water retention in the body, exacerbating swelling and oedema in individuals with lymphedema. Excessive sodium intake can disrupt the body's fluid balance, increasing fluid accumulation in the affected areas and causing discomfort and tightness. Therefore, reducing sodium intake through minimizing processed foods, avoiding added salt, and opting for fresh, whole foods can help alleviate swelling and discomfort associated with lymphedema.

2. **Fluid Intake**: Proper hydration is essential for lymphedema management, as adequate fluid intake helps maintain lymphatic function and supports the body's ability to flush out toxins and excess fluid. However, excessive fluid intake can also contribute to swelling in individuals with lymphedema. It's important to strike a balance by consuming enough fluids to stay hydrated without overloading the lymphatic system. Monitoring fluid intake and spreading it out throughout the day can help prevent fluid buildup and reduce swelling.

3. **Inflammatory Foods**: Certain foods can trigger inflammation in the body, exacerbating lymphedema symptoms such as swelling and discomfort. These inflammatory foods may include processed foods, refined sugars, trans fats, and foods high in omega-6 fatty acids. Consuming a diet rich in anti-inflammatory foods, such as fruits, vegetables, whole grains, and omega-3 fatty acids, can help reduce inflammation and alleviate lymphedema symptoms.

4. **Weight Management**: Maintaining a healthy weight is crucial for managing lymphedema, as excess body weight can put additional strain on the lymphatic system and exacerbate swelling and discomfort. Adopting a balanced diet that supports weight management, including portion control, nutrient-dense foods, and regular physical activity, can help prevent further progression of lymphedema and improve mobility and comfort.

FOODS TO INCLUDE

1. **High-Fiber Foods**: Whole grains, legumes, fruits, and vegetables help maintain bowel regularity and prevent constipation, which can exacerbate lymphedema symptoms.

2. **Lean Protein Sources**: Skinless poultry, fish, tofu, beans, and legumes provide essential amino acids for tissue repair and maintenance without excess saturated fat.

3. **Healthy Fats**: Incorporate sources of healthy fats such as avocados, nuts, seeds, and olive oil to support overall health and reduce inflammation.

4. **Fresh Fruits and Vegetables:** Opt for a variety of colourful fruits and vegetables rich in antioxidants and vitamins to support immune function and reduce inflammation.

5. **Hydrating Foods:** Include foods with high water content such as cucumber, watermelon, strawberries, and leafy greens to support hydration and promote healthy lymphatic flow.

6. **Herbs and Spices**: Incorporate herbs and spices like ginger, turmeric, garlic, and cinnamon known for their anti-inflammatory properties.

7. **Low-Sodium Options:** Choose low-sodium alternatives to minimize fluid retention, including fresh foods over processed options and seasoning dishes with herbs and spices instead of salt. Example: Fresh fruits and vegetables, unsalted nuts, homemade meals with minimal added salt.

8. **Hydration:** Drink plenty of water throughout the day to support lymphatic drainage and overall hydration.

FOODS TO AVOID

1. **High-Sodium Foods**: Minimize intake of processed and packaged foods, canned soups, deli meats, and salty snacks, as excess sodium can contribute to fluid retention.

2. **Processed Foods**: Avoid processed and refined foods such as sugary snacks, white bread, pastries, and fried foods, which can promote inflammation and hinder lymphatic function.

3. **High-Sugar Foods:** Limit consumption of sugary beverages, candies, desserts, and sweetened snacks, as excessive sugar intake can exacerbate inflammation and compromise immune function.

4. **Alcohol**: Reduce alcohol consumption, as it can dehydrate the body and impair lymphatic function.

5. **Trans Fats:** Avoid foods high in trans fats, such as fried foods, processed snacks, and baked goods, as they can promote inflammation and contribute to overall health issues.

6. **Excessive Caffeine**: Limit intake of caffeinated beverages, as they can have a diuretic effect and potentially exacerbate dehydration.

7. **Allergenic Foods**: If you have known food sensitivities or allergies, avoid triggering foods that may exacerbate inflammation and worsen lymphedema symptoms.

8. **Large Meals**: Instead of consuming large meals, opt for smaller, more frequent meals throughout the day to avoid overloading the lymphatic system.

Chapter 2
Breakfast Recipes

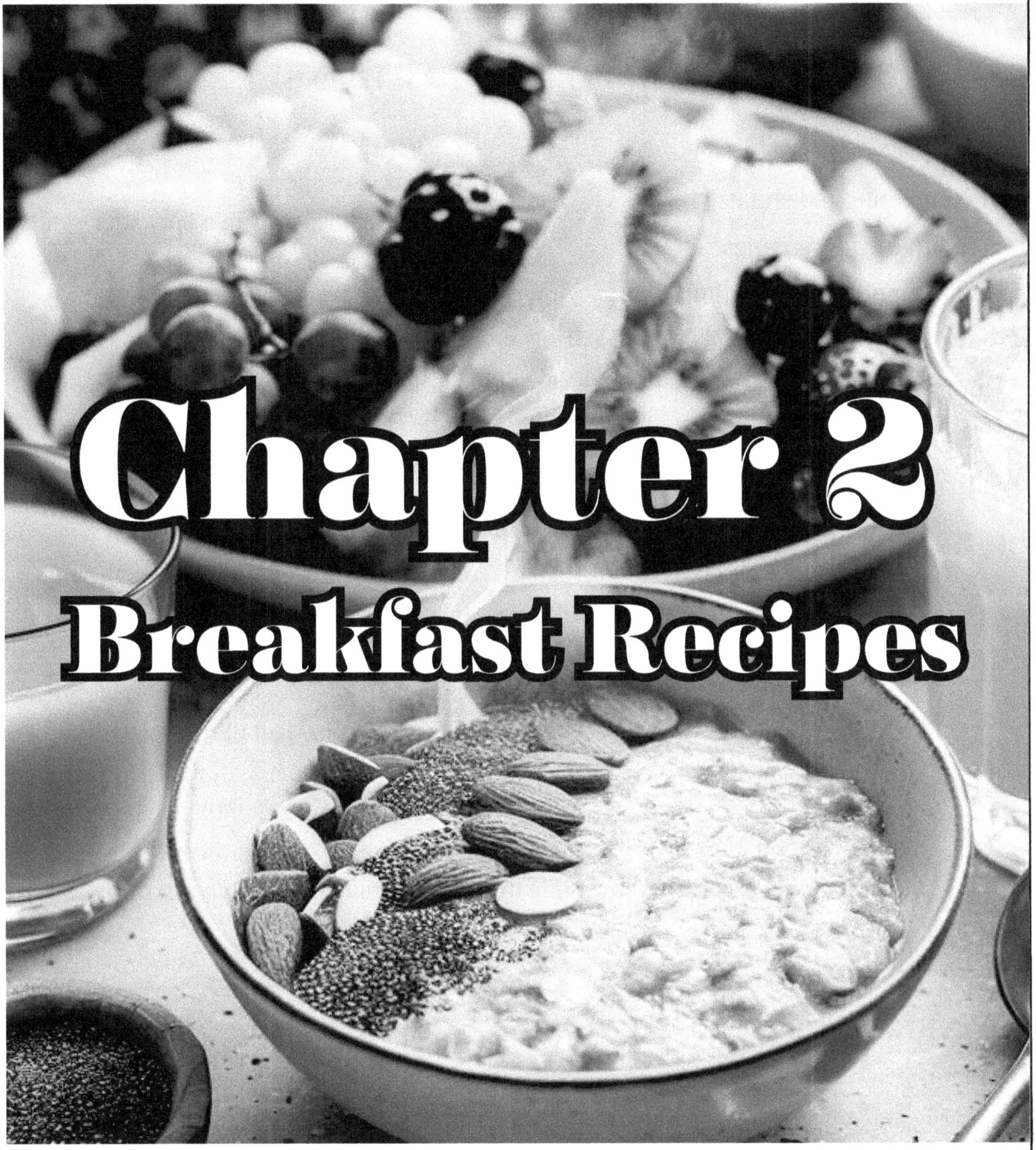

Veggie Omelette with Spinach and Tomatoes

 2 servings  10 minutes

INGREDIENTS

2 large eggs

1/4 cup chopped spinach

1/4 cup diced tomatoes

2 tablespoons diced onion

1/4 cup shredded cheese
(optional)

Salt and pepper to taste

1 teaspoon olive oil or
cooking spray

DIRECTIONS

1. In a small bowl, beat the eggs until well-mixed. Season with salt and pepper.
2. Heat olive oil or cooking spray in a non-stick skillet over medium heat.
3. Add diced onion to the skillet and cook until translucent, about 2 minutes.
4. Add chopped spinach and diced tomatoes to the skillet. Cook for an additional 2 minutes, until spinach is wilted and tomatoes are softened.
5. Pour the beaten eggs evenly over the vegetables in the skillet.
6. Cook the omelette for 2-3 minutes, lifting the edges with a spatula and tilting the skillet to let uncooked eggs flow underneath.
7. Once the omelette is mostly set, sprinkle shredded cheese (if using) over one-half of the omelette.
8. Carefully fold the omelette in half with a spatula and cook for another 1-2 minutes, until the cheese is melted and the eggs are cooked through.
9. Slide the omelette onto a plate and serve hot.

NUTRITION INFO

Calories: 150 kcal

Protein: 12g

Fat: 9g

Carbohydrates: 6g

Fiber: 2g

Sugar: 3g

Sodium: 170mg

Buckwheat Pancakes with Greek Yogurt and Honey

 4 servings  25 minutes

INGREDIENTS

1 cup buckwheat flour

1 tablespoon baking powder

1/4 teaspoon salt

1 tablespoon honey

1 cup almond milk (or any milk of your choice)

1 large egg

1 tablespoon melted coconut oil (plus extra for cooking)

Greek yogurt, for serving

Honey, for drizzling

DIRECTIONS

1. In a large mixing bowl, whisk together the buckwheat flour, baking powder, and salt.
2. In another bowl, whisk together the honey, almond milk, egg, and melted coconut oil until well combined.
3. Pour the wet ingredients into the dry ingredients and stir until just combined. Do not overmix; a few lumps are okay.
4. Heat a non-stick skillet or griddle over medium heat and lightly grease with coconut oil.
5. Pour about 1/4 cup of batter onto the skillet for each pancake. Cook until bubbles form on the surface, then flip and cook until golden brown on the other side, about 2-3 minutes per side.
6. Repeat with the remaining batter, greasing the skillet as needed.
7. Serve the pancakes warm, topped with a dollop of Greek yogurt and a drizzle of honey.

NUTRITION INFO

Calories: 220 kcal

Protein: 7g

Carbohydrates: 32g

Fat: 7g

Fiber: 4g

Sugar: 6g

Sodium: 430mg

Chia Seed Pudding with Fresh Fruit

 2 servings

 5 minutes

INGREDIENTS

1/4 cup chia seeds

1 cup almond milk (or any milk of your choice)

1 tablespoon maple syrup or honey (optional, adjust to taste)

1/2 teaspoon vanilla extract

Fresh fruit (such as berries, sliced banana, mango, or kiwi) for topping

DIRECTIONS

1. In a mixing bowl or jar, combine chia seeds, almond milk, maple syrup (if using), and vanilla extract.
2. Stir well to combine, ensuring there are no clumps of chia seeds.
3. Cover the bowl or jar and refrigerate for at least 2 hours, or preferably overnight, to allow the chia seeds to gel and thicken.
4. Once the chia pudding has set, give it a good stir to evenly distribute the seeds.
5. Divide the chia pudding into serving bowls or glasses.
6. Top with your favorite fresh fruit.
7. Serve chilled and enjoy!

NUTRITION INFO

Calories: 150 kcal Total

Total Fat: 7g   Carbohydrates: 19g

Saturated Fat: 0.5g Dietary Fiber: 10g

Cholesterol: 0mg Sugars: 6g

Sodium: 80mg   Protein: 4g

Quinoa Breakfast Porridge with Berries

 2 servings

 25 minutes

INGREDIENTS

1/2 cup quinoa, rinsed

1 cup almond milk (or any milk of your choice)

1/2 teaspoon ground cinnamon

1/4 teaspoon vanilla extract

Pinch of salt

1/2 cup mixed berries (such as strawberries, blueberries, raspberries)

2 tablespoons chopped nuts (such as almonds, walnuts, or pecans)

1 tablespoon honey or maple syrup (optional, for sweetness)

DIRECTIONS

1. In a small saucepan, combine the quinoa and almond milk. Bring to a boil over medium heat.
2. Reduce the heat to low and simmer, covered, for about 15 minutes, or until the quinoa is cooked and the liquid is absorbed. Stir occasionally.
3. Stir in the ground cinnamon, vanilla extract, and a pinch of salt.
4. Remove the saucepan from the heat and let the quinoa porridge cool slightly.
5. Divide the quinoa porridge into serving bowls.
6. Top each bowl with mixed berries and chopped nuts.
7. Drizzle with honey or maple syrup for added sweetness, if desired.
8. Serve warm and enjoy!

NUTRITION INFO

Calories: 250	Total
Total Fat: 7g	Carbohydrates: 40g
Saturated Fat: 0.5g	Dietary Fiber: 5g
Cholesterol: 0mg	Sugars: 10g
Sodium: 80mg	Protein: 7g

Green Smoothie Bowl

 2 servings  10 minutes

INGREDIENTS

2 cups fresh spinach leaves

1 ripe banana, frozen

1 cup frozen mango chunks

1/2 ripe avocado

1/2 cup unsweetened almond milk (or any milk of choice)

1 tablespoon chia seeds

Toppings (optional):

    Sliced kiwi

    Sliced strawberries

    Granola

    Unsweetened shredded coconut

    Chia seeds

    Honey or maple syrup (optional)

DIRECTIONS

1. In a blender, combine the spinach, frozen banana, frozen mango, avocado, almond milk, and chia seeds.
2. Blend on high until smooth and creamy, adding more almond milk if needed to reach your desired consistency.
3. Pour the smoothie into bowls.
4. Top with sliced kiwi, sliced strawberries, granola, shredded coconut, and additional chia seeds if desired.
5. Drizzle with honey or maple syrup for added sweetness, if desired.
6. Serve immediately and enjoy your nutritious green smoothie bowl!

NUTRITION INFO

Calories: 250	Total
Total Fat: 10g	Carbohydrates: 35g
Saturated Fat: 1.5g	Dietary Fiber: 8g
Cholesterol: 0mg	Sugars: 18g
Sodium: 80mg	Protein: 7g

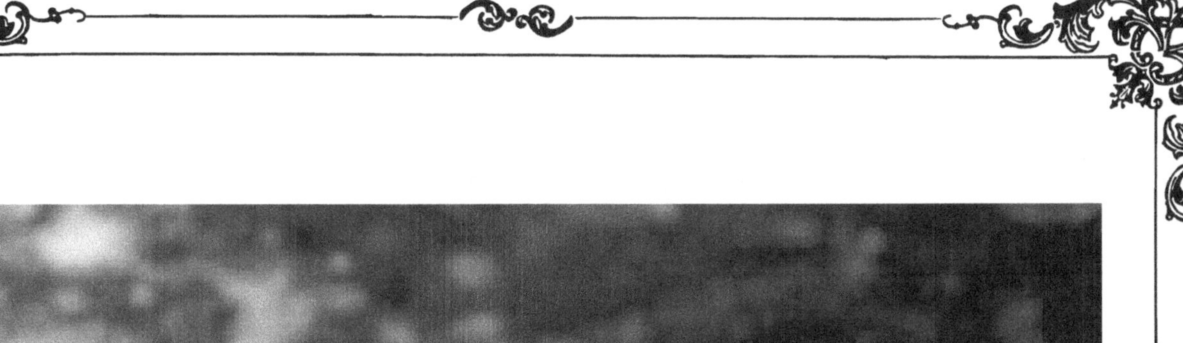
Chapter 3
Lunch Recipes

Grilled Chicken Salad with Avocado Dressing

4 servings

20 minutes

INGREDIENTS

2 boneless, skinless chicken breasts

6 cups mixed salad greens (lettuce, spinach, arugula, etc.)

1 cup cherry tomatoes, halved

1 cucumber, sliced

1/4 red onion, thinly sliced

1 avocado, diced

1/4 cup sliced almonds, toasted (optional)

Salt and pepper to taste

For the Avocado Dressing:

1 ripe avocado

1/4 cup Greek yogurt

2 tablespoons fresh lemon juice

2 tablespoons olive oil

1 garlic clove, minced

2 tablespoons chopped fresh cilantro or parsley

DIRECTIONS

1. Preheat the grill to medium-high heat. Season chicken breasts with salt and pepper. Grill chicken for 6-8 minutes per side, or until cooked through. Remove from grill and let rest for a few minutes before slicing.
2. Meanwhile, prepare the salad ingredients. In a large bowl, combine mixed salad greens, cherry tomatoes, cucumber slices, red onion slices, diced avocado, and toasted sliced almonds (if using).
3. To make the avocado dressing, combine the avocado, Greek yoghurt, lemon juice, olive oil, minced garlic, chopped cilantro or parsley, salt, and pepper in a blender or food processor. Blend until smooth. If the dressing is too thick, add water, 1 tablespoon at a time, until the desired consistency is reached.
4. Slice grilled chicken breasts and arrange them over the salad.
5. Drizzle the avocado dressing over the salad or serve on the side.
6. Toss the salad gently to coat with the dressing.
7. Serve immediately and enjoy!

NUTRITION INFO

Calories: 320

Protein: 25g

Carbohydrates: 14g

Fat: 20g

Fiber: 8g

Sugar: 3g

Sodium: 140mg

Lentil and Vegetable Soup

 4 servings    30minutes

INGREDIENTS

1 cup dry brown lentils, rinsed and drained
4 cups vegetable broth
1 tablespoon olive oil
1 onion, chopped
2 cloves garlic, minced
2 carrots, diced
2 celery stalks, diced
1 teaspoon ground cumin
1 teaspoon ground coriander
1/2 teaspoon smoked paprika
Salt and pepper to taste
1 can (14 oz) diced tomatoes
2 cups chopped spinach or kale
Juice of 1 lemon
Fresh parsley, for garnish (optional)

DIRECTIONS

1. In a large pot, heat the olive oil over medium heat. Add the chopped onion, garlic, carrots, and celery. Sauté until the vegetables are softened, about 5-7 minutes.
2. Add the ground cumin, ground coriander, smoked paprika, salt, and pepper. Stir well to coat the vegetables with the spices.
3. Add the rinsed lentils, vegetable broth, and diced tomatoes to the pot. Bring the soup to a boil, then reduce the heat to low and let it simmer for about 20-25 minutes, or until the lentils are tender.
4. Stir in the chopped spinach or kale and let it cook for an additional 5 minutes until wilted.
5. Remove the pot from the heat and stir in the lemon juice. Taste and adjust seasoning if needed.
6. Serve hot, garnished with fresh parsley if desired.

NUTRITION INFO

Calories: 235 kcal	Total Carbohydrates: 38 g
Total Fat: 4.5 g	
Saturated Fat: 0.6 g	Dietary Fiber: 15 g
Cholesterol: 0 mg	Sugars: 6 g
Sodium: 630 mg	Protein: 13 g

Turkey and Hummus Wrap with Mixed Greens

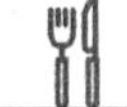 2 servings 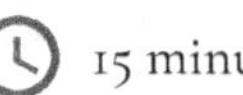 15 minutes

INGREDIENTS

4 large whole grain tortillas

8 oz (225g) sliced turkey breast

1/2 cup hummus

2 cups mixed salad greens

1 medium tomato, thinly sliced

1/2 cucumber, thinly sliced

1/4 red onion, thinly sliced

Salt and pepper to taste

DIRECTIONS

1. Lay out the tortillas on a clean work surface.
2. Spread 2 tablespoons of hummus evenly over each tortilla.
3. Divide the sliced turkey breast evenly among the tortillas, placing it in a single layer on top of the hummus.
4. Arrange the mixed salad greens, tomato slices, cucumber slices, and red onion slices over the turkey.
5. Season with salt and pepper to taste.
6. Roll up each tortilla tightly, folding in the sides as you go to enclose the filling.
7. Slice each wrap in half diagonally and serve immediately, or wrap tightly in plastic wrap for later consumption.

NUTRITION INFO

Calories: 320 kcal

Protein: 25g

Carbohydrates: 25g

Fiber: 6g

Fat: 12g

Saturated Fat: 2g

Cholesterol: 30mg

Sodium: 580mg

Salmon Nicoise Salad

 4 servings  25 minutes

INGREDIENTS

4 salmon fillets (about 4 ounces each)

1 pound small red potatoes, halved

4 large eggs

1/2 pound green beans, trimmed

2 cups cherry tomatoes, halved

1/2 cup Kalamata olives, pitted

4 cups mixed salad greens

1/4 cup red onion, thinly sliced

2 tablespoons capers

Salt and black pepper to taste

For the Dressing:

1/4 cup extra virgin olive oil

2 tablespoons red wine vinegar

1 teaspoon Dijon mustard

1 garlic clove, minced

1 tablespoon fresh lemon juice

DIRECTIONS

1. Preheat the oven to 400°F (200°C). Line a baking sheet with parchment paper.
2. Place the salmon fillets on one side of the baking sheet. Season with salt and pepper. Bake for 12-15 minutes, or until the salmon is cooked through and flakes easily with a fork.
3. While the salmon is baking, bring a large pot of salted water to a boil. Add the potatoes and cook for 10-12 minutes, or until tender. Drain and set aside.
4. In the same pot of boiling water, add the eggs and cook for 8-10 minutes for hard-boiled eggs. Once cooked, transfer the eggs to a bowl of ice water to cool. Once cooled, peel and quarter the eggs.
5. In another pot of boiling water, blanch the green beans for 2-3 minutes, then transfer them to a bowl of ice water to stop the cooking process. Drain and set aside.
6. In a small bowl, whisk together the ingredients for the dressing: olive oil, red wine vinegar, Dijon mustard, minced garlic, lemon juice, salt, and pepper.
7. Arrange the salad greens on a large serving platter. Top with cooked salmon, potatoes, hard-boiled eggs, blanched green beans, cherry tomatoes, Kalamata olives, red onion slices, and capers.
8. Drizzle the dressing over the salad or serve it on the side.
9. Season the salad with additional salt and pepper, if desired.
10. Serve immediately and enjoy!

NUTRITION INFO

Calories: 420 kcal

Total Fat: 24g

Saturated Fat: 4g

Trans Fat: 0g

Cholesterol: 160mg

Sodium: 560mg

Total Carbohydrates: 22g

Dietary Fiber: 4g

Sugars: 4g

Protein: 30g

Quinoa and Black Bean Stuffed Bell Peppers

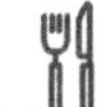 4 servings  45 minutes

INGREDIENTS

4 large bell peppers (any color)

1 cup quinoa, rinsed

1 can (15 oz) black beans, drained and rinsed

1 cup corn kernels (fresh, canned, or frozen)

1 cup diced tomatoes

1/2 cup diced onion

2 cloves garlic, minced

1 teaspoon ground cumin

1 teaspoon chili powder

Salt and pepper to taste

1 cup shredded cheese (cheddar or Mexican blend), optional

Fresh cilantro or parsley, for garnish (optional)

Olive oil, for drizzling

DIRECTIONS

1. Preheat your oven to 375°F (190°C). Grease a baking dish with olive oil or cooking spray.
2. Cut the tops off the bell peppers and remove the seeds and membranes. Place the peppers upright in the prepared baking dish.
3. In a medium saucepan, cook quinoa according to package instructions. Usually, this involves combining 1 cup quinoa with 2 cups water, bringing to a boil, then reducing heat and simmering for 15-20 minutes until the water is absorbed and the quinoa is fluffy.
4. In a large skillet, heat olive oil over medium heat. Add diced onion and minced garlic, and sauté until softened, about 3-4 minutes.
5. Add black beans, corn kernels, diced tomatoes, cooked quinoa, ground cumin, chili powder, salt, and pepper to the skillet. Stir well to combine and cook for another 5 minutes until heated through and flavors are well blended. Adjust seasoning to taste.
6. Spoon the quinoa and black bean mixture evenly into each bell pepper, packing it down gently. If using cheese, sprinkle it over the top of each stuffed pepper.
7. Cover the baking dish with foil and bake in the preheated oven for 25-30 minutes, or until the peppers are tender.
8. Remove the foil and bake for an additional 5 minutes, or until the cheese is melted and bubbly (if using).
9. Once done, remove from the oven and let cool slightly before serving. Garnish with fresh cilantro or parsley if desired.

NUTRITION INFO

Calories: 305 kcal

Protein: 11g

Carbohydrates: 55g

Fat: 4g

Fiber: 11g

Sugar: 7g

Sodium: 384mg

Chapter 4
Snack Recipes

Edamame and Roasted Chickpea Mix

★★★★★

 1 servings 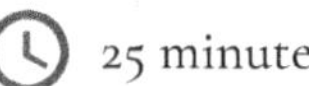 25 minutes

INGREDIENTS

1 cup cooked edamame (shelled)

1 cup cooked chickpeas (drained and rinsed if using canned)

1 tablespoon olive oil

1 teaspoon garlic powder

1 teaspoon paprika

1/2 teaspoon cumin

Salt and pepper to taste

DIRECTIONS

1. Preheat your oven to 400°F (200°C) and line a baking sheet with parchment paper.
2. In a bowl, combine the cooked edamame and chickpeas.
3. Drizzle the olive oil over the edamame and chickpeas, then sprinkle with garlic powder, paprika, cumin, salt, and pepper. Toss until evenly coated.
4. Spread the seasoned edamame and chickpeas in a single layer on the prepared baking sheet.
5. Roast in the preheated oven for 20-25 minutes, stirring halfway through, until the chickpeas are crispy and golden brown.
6. Remove from the oven and let cool slightly before serving.

NUTRITION INFO

Calories: 220 kcal

Protein: 12g

Carbohydrates: 25g

Fiber: 8g

Sugars: 4g

Fat: 9g

Saturated Fat: 1g

Sodium: 15mg

Greek Yogurt with Berries and Almonds

 1 servings  5 minutes

INGREDIENTS

1/2 cup Greek yogurt

1/4 cup mixed berries (such as strawberries, blueberries, raspberries)

1 tablespoon sliced almonds

1 teaspoon honey (optional, for added sweetness)

DIRECTIONS

1. Spoon Greek yoghurt into a serving bowl or glass.
2. Wash and prepare the mixed berries, then place them on top of the yoghurt.
3. Sprinkle sliced almonds over the berries.
4. Drizzle honey over the top, if desired, for added sweetness.
5. Serve immediately and enjoy!

NUTRITION INFO

Calories: Approximately 180 kcal

Protein: Approximately 15g

Fat: Approximately 7g

Carbohydrates: Approximately 15g

Fiber: Approximately 3g

Sugars: Approximately 10g

Vegetable Crudité with Hummus

 4 servings  15 minutes

INGREDIENTS

2 large carrots, peeled and cut into sticks

2 cucumbers, sliced

2 bell peppers (red, yellow, or green), sliced

1 cup cherry tomatoes

1 cup snap peas

1 cup broccoli florets

1 cup cauliflower florets

1 cup hummus (store-bought or homemade)

Fresh parsley or dill for garnish (optional)

DIRECTIONS

1. Wash and prepare all the vegetables as needed. Arrange them on a serving platter or individual plates.
2. Place the hummus in a bowl and garnish with fresh parsley or dill if desired.
3. Serve the vegetable crudité alongside the hummus for dipping.

NUTRITION INFO

Calories: 150

Total Fat: 7g

Saturated Fat: 1g

Trans Fat: 0g

Cholesterol: 0mg

Sodium: 250mg

Total Carbohydrates: 19g

Dietary Fiber: 7g

Sugars: 6g

Protein: 6g

Cottage Cheese and Pineapple Cups

 4 servings    15 minutes

INGREDIENTS

1 cup cottage cheese

1 cup diced pineapple (fresh or canned in juice, drained)

2 tablespoons honey (optional)

1 teaspoon vanilla extract

1/4 cup chopped walnuts or almonds (optional)

Fresh mint leaves for garnish (optional)

DIRECTIONS

1. In a mixing bowl, combine cottage cheese, diced pineapple, honey (if using), and vanilla extract. Stir well to combine.
2. Divide the mixture evenly into 4 serving cups or bowls.
3. If desired, sprinkle chopped walnuts or almonds over the top of each cup.
4. Garnish with fresh mint leaves for a burst of color and flavor.
5. Serve immediately, or refrigerate until ready to enjoy.

NUTRITION INFO

Calories: 150 kcal

Protein: 13g

Carbohydrates: 14g

Fat: 5g

Fiber: 1g

Sugar: 12g

Sodium: 250mg

Rice Cake with Almond Butter and Banana Slices

1 servings

5 minutes

INGREDIENTS

1 rice cake

1 tablespoon almond butter

1/2 ripe banana, sliced

Optional: drizzle of honey or sprinkle of cinnamon for added flavor

DIRECTIONS

1. Spread almond butter evenly on top of the rice cake.
2. Arrange banana slices on top of the almond butter layer.
3. Optional: Drizzle honey or sprinkle cinnamon over the banana slices for added sweetness or flavour.
4. Serve immediately and enjoy!

NUTRITION INFO

Calories: 150 kcal

Total Fat: 7g

Saturated Fat: 1g

Trans Fat: 0g

Cholesterol: 0mg

Sodium: 70mg

Total Carbohydrates: 20g

Dietary Fiber: 3g

Sugars: 6g

Protein: 4g

Chapter 5
Dinner Recipes

Baked Cod with Lemon and Dill

 4 servings  20 minutes

INGREDIENTS

4 cod fillets (about 6 ounces each)

2 tablespoons olive oil

2 tablespoons freshly squeezed lemon juice

2 cloves garlic, minced

1 tablespoon fresh dill, chopped

Salt and pepper to taste

Lemon slices for garnish

Fresh dill sprigs for garnish

DIRECTIONS

1. Preheat your oven to 375°F (190°C). Lightly grease a baking dish with olive oil or cooking spray.
2. Rinse the cod fillets under cold water and pat them dry with paper towels. Place them in the prepared baking dish, leaving space between each fillet.
3. In a small bowl, whisk together the olive oil, lemon juice, minced garlic, and chopped dill. Season the mixture with salt and pepper to taste.
4. Pour the lemon-dill mixture over the cod fillets, making sure each fillet is evenly coated.
5. Place a few lemon slices on top of each fillet for extra flavor.
6. Bake the cod in the preheated oven for about 15-20 minutes, or until the fish is opaque and flakes easily with a fork.
7. Once cooked, remove the cod from the oven and let it rest for a few minutes before serving.
8. Garnish with fresh dill sprigs before serving. Enjoy your baked cod with lemon and dill!

NUTRITION INFO

Calories: 180 kcal

Protein: 25g

Fat: 7g

Carbohydrates: 3g

Fiber: 1g

Sodium: 240mg

Spaghetti Squash with Turkey Bolognese Sauce

★★★★★

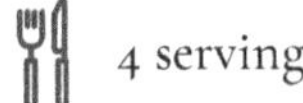 4 servings

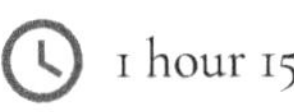 1 hour 15 minutes

INGREDIENTS

1 medium spaghetti squash

1 tablespoon olive oil

1 pound lean ground turkey

1 onion, fincly chopped

2 cloves garlic, minced

1 can (14 oz) crushed tomatoes

1 tablespoon tomato paste

1 teaspoon dried oregano

1 teaspoon dried basil

Salt and pepper, to taste

Fresh parsley, chopped (for garnish)

Grated Parmesan cheese (optional, for serving)

DIRECTIONS

1. Preheat your oven to 400°F (200°C).
2. Carefully cut the spaghetti squash in half lengthwise and scoop out the seeds with a spoon.
3. Drizzle the cut sides of the squash with olive oil and season with salt and pepper.
4. Place the squash halves, cut side down, on a baking sheet lined with parchment paper.
5. Roast in the preheated oven for about 40-45 minutes, or until the squash is tender and the flesh easily shreds into strands with a fork.
6. While the squash is roasting, heat olive oil in a large skillet over medium heat. Add the chopped onion and cook until softened, about 3-4 minutes. Add the minced garlic and cook for another minute.
7. Add the ground turkey to the skillet and cook until browned, breaking it up with a spoon as it cooks.
8. Stir in the crushed tomatoes, tomato paste, dried oregano, and dried basil. Season with salt and pepper to taste. Simmer the sauce for about 10-15 minutes, allowing the flavors to meld.
9. Once the squash is cooked, use a fork to scrape the flesh into strands.
10. Serve the spaghetti squash topped with the turkey Bolognese sauce. Garnish with chopped parsley and grated Parmesan cheese if desired.

NUTRITION INFO

Calories: 280 kcal

Total Fat: 10g

Saturated Fat: 2g

Cholesterol: 60mg

Sodium: 380mg

Total Carbohydrates: 22g

Dietary Fiber: 5g

Sugars: 9g

Protein: 25g

Stir-fried tofu with Broccoli and Brown Rice

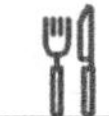

★★★★★

4 servings   35 minutes

INGREDIENTS

1 block (14 oz) firm tofu, drained and pressed
2 cups broccoli florets
1 red bell pepper, thinly sliced
3 cloves garlic, minced
1 tablespoon ginger, minced
2 tablespoons low-sodium soy sauce
1 tablespoon sesame oil
1 tablespoon rice vinegar
2 tablespoons vegetable oil, divided
4 cups cooked brown rice
Salt and pepper to taste
Optional garnish: sesame seeds, chopped green onions

DIRECTIONS

1. Prepare Tofu: Cut the tofu into cubes and pat dry with paper towels to remove excess moisture. Season with salt and pepper to taste.
2. Stir-fry Tofu: Heat 1 tablespoon of vegetable oil in a large skillet or wok over medium-high heat. Add the tofu cubes and cook until golden brown on all sides, about 5-7 minutes. Remove tofu from the skillet and set aside.
3. Cook Vegetables: In the same skillet, add the remaining tablespoon of vegetable oil. Add minced garlic and ginger, stirring constantly for about 30 seconds until fragrant. Add broccoli florets and sliced bell pepper to the skillet. Stir-fry for 3-4 minutes until the vegetables are tender-crisp.
4. Combine Ingredients: Return the cooked tofu to the skillet with the vegetables. Add soy sauce, sesame oil, and rice vinegar. Stir well to combine all ingredients evenly. Cook for an additional 2-3 minutes, allowing the flavors to meld.
5. Serve: Serve the stir-fried tofu and broccoli over cooked brown rice. Garnish with sesame seeds and chopped green onions if desired.

NUTRITION INFO

Calories: 320 kcal
Protein: 14g
Fat: 14g
Carbohydrates: 36g
Fiber: 6g
Sugar: 3g
Sodium: 480mg

Grilled Vegetable and Quinoa Salad

 4 servings    30 minutes

INGREDIENTS

1 cup quinoa, rinsed

2 cups water or vegetable broth

1 red bell pepper, sliced

1 yellow bell pepper, sliced

1 zucchini, sliced lengthwise

1 yellow squash, sliced lengthwise

1 small red onion, sliced into rings

1 cup cherry tomatoes, halved

2 tablespoons olive oil

Salt and pepper to taste

2 tablespoons balsamic vinegar

2 tablespoons fresh lemon juice

1 garlic clove, minced

2 tablespoons fresh basil, chopped

Optional: crumbled feta cheese or goat cheese for topping

DIRECTIONS

1. In a medium saucepan, combine quinoa and water or vegetable broth. Bring to a boil, then reduce heat to low, cover, and simmer for 15-20 minutes, or until quinoa is cooked and water is absorbed. Remove from heat and let it cool.
2. Preheat grill or grill pan over medium-high heat.
3. In a large bowl, toss the sliced bell peppers, zucchini, yellow squash, and red onion with olive oil, salt, and pepper.
4. Grill the vegetables for 3-4 minutes per side, or until they are tender and have grill marks. Remove from the grill and let them cool slightly.
5. In a small bowl, whisk together balsamic vinegar, lemon juice, minced garlic, and chopped basil to make the dressing.
6. In a large serving bowl, combine cooked quinoa, grilled vegetables, cherry tomatoes, and dressing. Toss gently to coat everything evenly.
7. Serve the salad at room temperature or chilled, topped with crumbled feta cheese or goat cheese if desired.

NUTRITION INFO

Calories: 280 kcal

Total Fat: 10g

Saturated Fat: 2g

Trans Fat: 0g

Cholesterol: 0mg

Sodium: 120mg

Total Carbohydrates: 40g

Dietary Fiber: 6g

Sugars: 6g

Protein: 8g

Chicken Stir-Fry with Snow Peas and Cashews

★★★★★

 4 servings  30 minutes

INGREDIENTS

1 lb (450g) boneless, skinless chicken breasts, thinly sliced

2 tablespoons soy sauce (low-sodium if preferred)

2 tablespoons oyster sauce

1 tablespoon rice vinegar

1 tablespoon sesame oil

2 cloves garlic, minced

1 teaspoon fresh ginger, grated

1 tablespoon cornstarch

2 tablespoons vegetable oil

2 cups (200g) snow peas, ends trimmed

1 red bell pepper, thinly sliced

1/2 cup (50g) unsalted cashews

Cooked rice or noodles, for serving

Sliced green onions and sesame seeds, for garnish (optional)

DIRECTIONS

1. In a small bowl, whisk together soy sauce, oyster sauce, rice vinegar, sesame oil, minced garlic, grated ginger, and cornstarch. Set aside.
2. Heat vegetable oil in a large skillet or wok over medium-high heat. Add sliced chicken and cook until browned and cooked through, about 5-6 minutes. Remove chicken from the skillet and set aside.
3. In the same skillet, add snow peas and sliced red bell pepper. Stir-fry for 2-3 minutes until vegetables are tender-crisp.
4. Return the cooked chicken to the skillet. Pour the sauce over the chicken and vegetables, stirring well to coat everything evenly. Cook for another 2-3 minutes until the sauce has thickened.
5. Add unsalted cashews to the skillet and toss to combine.
6. Serve the chicken stir-fry hot over cooked rice or noodles. Garnish with sliced green onions and sesame seeds, if desired.

NUTRITION INFO

Calories: 350 kcal

Protein: 28g

Carbohydrates: 16g

Fat: 20g

Fiber: 3g

Sugar: 4g

Sodium: 650mg

CHAPTER 6

Dessert Recipes

Berry Parfait with Greek Yogurt and Granola

 1 servings   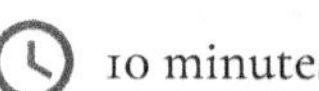 10 minutes

INGREDIENTS

1/2 cup Greek yogurt (unsweetened)

1/4 cup mixed berries (such as strawberries, blueberries, raspberries)

1/4 cup granola (choose a low-sugar or homemade option for healthier choice)

1 teaspoon honey (optional, for drizzling)

DIRECTIONS

1. In a glass or parfait dish, spoon a layer of Greek yogurt into the bottom.
2. Add a layer of mixed berries on top of the yogurt.
3. Sprinkle a layer of granola over the berries.
4. Repeat the layers until the glass is filled, ending with a sprinkle of granola on top.
5. If desired, drizzle honey over the top for added sweetness.
6. Serve immediately and enjoy!

NUTRITION INFO

Calories: 250 kcal

Protein: 15g

Carbohydrates: 30g

Fat: 8g

Fiber: 5g

Sugar: 15g (may vary depending on yogurt and granola used)

Calcium: 15% DV

Vitamin C: 20% DV

Dark Chocolate Avocado Mousse

 4 servings  15 minutes

INGREDIENTS

2 ripe avocados

1/4 cup unsweetened cocoa powder

1/4 cup maple syrup or honey (adjust to taste)

1 teaspoon vanilla extract

Pinch of salt

Optional toppings: fresh berries, shaved dark chocolate, whipped cream

DIRECTIONS

1. Cut the avocados in half, remove the pits, and scoop the flesh into a blender or food processor.
2. Add cocoa powder, maple syrup or honey, vanilla extract, and a pinch of salt to the blender or food processor.
3. Blend until smooth and creamy, scraping down the sides as needed to ensure all ingredients are well incorporated.
4. Taste and adjust sweetness as desired by adding more maple syrup or honey.
5. Transfer the mousse to serving dishes or glasses.
6. Chill in the refrigerator for at least 30 minutes before serving.
7. Garnish with fresh berries, shaved dark chocolate, or whipped cream if desired.
8. Serve chilled and enjoy!

NUTRITION INFO

Calories: 200 kcal

Total Fat: 15g

Saturated Fat: 2g

Sodium: 5mg

Total Carbohydrates: 20g

Dietary Fiber: 8g

Sugars: 10g

Protein: 3g

Baked Apples with Cinnamon and Walnuts

 4 servings 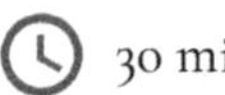 30 minutes

INGREDIENTS

4 large apples (such as Honeycrisp or Granny Smith)

1/4 cup chopped walnuts

2 tablespoons honey or maple syrup

1 teaspoon ground cinnamon

1/4 teaspoon ground nutmeg

1/4 teaspoon ground cloves

1 tablespoon lemon juice

1 tablespoon unsalted butter or coconut oil, melted

Optional: Vanilla Greek yogurt or vanilla ice cream for serving

DIRECTIONS

1. Preheat your oven to 375°F (190°C). Lightly grease a baking dish with butter or non-stick cooking spray.
2. Wash the apples thoroughly and pat them dry. Using an apple corer or a sharp knife, remove the cores from the apples, leaving the bottoms intact to create a well for the filling.
3. In a small bowl, mix together the chopped walnuts, honey or maple syrup, cinnamon, nutmeg, cloves, lemon juice, and melted butter or coconut oil until well combined.
4. Stuff each apple with the walnut mixture, dividing it evenly among the apples. Place the stuffed apples in the prepared baking dish.
5. Cover the baking dish with aluminum foil and bake in the preheated oven for 20 minutes.
6. After 20 minutes, remove the foil and continue baking for an additional 10-15 minutes, or until the apples are tender and the filling is bubbly.
7. Once baked, remove the apples from the oven and allow them to cool slightly before serving.
8. Serve the baked apples warm, optionally topped with a dollop of vanilla Greek yogurt or a scoop of vanilla ice cream.

NUTRITION INFO

Calories: 192 kcal

Total Fat: 7g

Saturated Fat: 2g

Cholesterol: 7mg

Sodium: 3mg

Total Carbohydrates: 35g

Dietary Fiber: 6g

Sugars: 26g

Protein: 1g

Frozen Banana Bites with Peanut Butter Drizzle

 4 servings  15 minutes

INGREDIENTS

2 ripe bananas

¼ cup creamy peanut butter

2 tablespoons dark chocolate chips

1 teaspoon coconut oil

Optional toppings: crushed nuts, shredded coconut, chia seeds

DIRECTIONS

1. Peel the bananas and cut them into thick slices, about 1/2 inch thick.
2. Place the banana slices on a baking sheet lined with parchment paper.
3. Insert a toothpick into each banana slice and freeze for at least 1 hour or until firm.
4. In a microwave-safe bowl, combine the peanut butter, dark chocolate chips, and coconut oil. Microwave in 20-second intervals, stirring in between, until melted and smooth.
5. Remove the frozen banana slices from the freezer and drizzle the peanut butter mixture over each slice using a spoon.
6. Sprinkle optional toppings over the banana bites if desired.
7. Return the banana bites to the freezer and freeze for an additional 30 minutes or until the peanut butter drizzle is set.
8. Serve immediately or store in an airtight container in the freezer for later enjoyment.

NUTRITION INFO

Calories: 160 kcal

Total Fat: 9g

Saturated Fat: 3g

Cholesterol: 0mg

Sodium: 75mg

Total Carbohydrates: 18g

Dietary Fiber: 3g

Sugars: 10g

Protein: 4g

Coconut Milk Rice Pudding with Mango

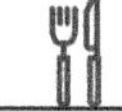 4 serving 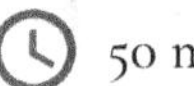 50 minutes

INGREDIENTS

1 cup jasmine rice

1 can (13.5 oz) coconut milk

2 cups water

1/4 cup sugar (adjust to taste)

1 teaspoon vanilla extract

1 ripe mango, diced

Toasted coconut flakes, for garnish (optional)

DIRECTIONS

1. Rinse the jasmine rice under cold water until the water runs clear. Drain excess water.
2. In a medium saucepan, combine the rinsed rice, coconut milk, water, and sugar. Stir well.
3. Bring the mixture to a boil over medium-high heat, then reduce the heat to low and simmer, uncovered, stirring occasionally, for about 30-35 minutes or until the rice is tender and the mixture has thickened to a pudding-like consistency.
4. Remove the saucepan from the heat and stir in the vanilla extract.
5. Let the rice pudding cool slightly before serving. Serve warm or chilled, topped with diced mango and toasted coconut flakes if desired.

NUTRITION INFO

Calories: 382 kcal

Fat: 19g

Saturated Fat: 17g

Carbohydrates: 51g

Sugar: 20g

Protein: 4g

Fiber: 2g

Sodium: 20mg

Chapter 7
Beverages and Smoothies

Green Detox Smoothie

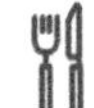 2 servings    5 minutes

INGREDIENTS

2 cups fresh spinach leaves

1 ripe banana, peeled and sliced

1 green apple, cored and chopped

1/2 cucumber, peeled and chopped

1/2 lemon, juiced

1 tablespoon fresh ginger, grated

1 cup coconut water or water

Ice cubes (optional)

DIRECTIONS

1. In a blender, combine the spinach leaves, banana, green apple, cucumber, lemon juice, and grated ginger.
2. Add the coconut water or water to the blender.
3. Blend on high speed until the mixture is smooth and well-combined. If desired, add ice cubes for a colder smoothie.
4. Pour the smoothie into glasses and serve immediately.
5. Enjoy this refreshing and nutritious green detox smoothie as part of your lymphedema-friendly diet.

NUTRITION INFO

Calories: 150

Total Fat: 1g

Saturated Fat: 0g

Cholesterol: 0mg

Sodium: 20mg

Total Carbohydrates: 35g

Dietary Fiber: 8g

Sugars: 20g

Protein: 5g

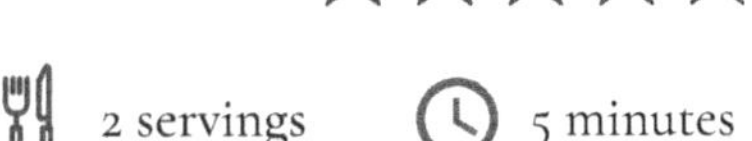

Green Detox Smoothie

2 servings · 5 minutes

INGREDIENTS

2 cups fresh spinach leaves

1 ripe banana, peeled and sliced

1 green apple, cored and chopped

1/2 cucumber, peeled and chopped

1/2 lemon, juiced

1 tablespoon fresh ginger, grated

1 cup coconut water or water

Ice cubes (optional)

DIRECTIONS

1. In a blender, combine the spinach leaves, banana, green apple, cucumber, lemon juice, and grated ginger.
2. Add the coconut water or water to the blender.
3. Blend on high speed until the mixture is smooth and well-combined. If desired, add ice cubes for a colder smoothie.
4. Pour the smoothie into glasses and serve immediately.
5. Enjoy this refreshing and nutritious green detox smoothie as part of your lymphedema-friendly diet.

NUTRITION INFO

Calories: 150	Total Carbohydrates: 35g
Total Fat: 1g	
Saturated Fat: 0g	
Cholesterol: 0mg	Dietary Fiber: 8g
Sodium: 20mg	Sugars: 20g
	Protein: 5g

Herbal Iced Tea with Lemon and Mint

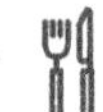 4 servings  10 minutes

INGREDIENTS

4 cups water

4 herbal tea bags (choose your favorite herbal blend)

1 lemon, thinly sliced

Handful of fresh mint leaves

Ice cubes, for serving

Lemon slices and mint sprigs, for garnish (optional)

DIRECTIONS

1. In a medium saucepan, bring the water to a boil.
2. Remove the saucepan from the heat and add the tea bags. Let steep for 5-7 minutes, depending on the strength of the tea desired.
3. Once steeped, remove the tea bags and discard them.
4. Allow the tea to cool to room temperature, then transfer it to a pitcher.
5. Add the lemon slices and fresh mint leaves to the pitcher.
6. Refrigerate the tea for at least 1 hour to chill and allow the flavours to meld.
7. To serve, fill glasses with ice cubes and pour the chilled tea over the ice.
8. Garnish each glass with a slice of lemon and a sprig of mint, if desired.
9. Enjoy your refreshing Herbal Iced Tea with Lemon and Mint!

NUTRITION INFO

Calories: 5

Total Fat: 0g

Cholesterol: 0mg

Sodium: 5mg

Total Carbohydrates: 1g

Dietary Fiber: 0g

Sugars: 0g

Protein: 0g

Protein-Packed Berry Smoothie

★★★★★

1 servings   5 min

INGREDIENTS

1 cup mixed berries (such as strawberries, blueberries, and raspberries), fresh or frozen

1/2 cup Greek yogurt (plain or flavored)

1/2 cup almond milk (or any milk of your choice)

1 scoop of your favorite protein powder (vanilla or berry-flavored)

1 tablespoon honey or maple syrup (optional, for sweetness)

Ice cubes (optional, for a colder smoothie)

DIRECTIONS

1. In a blender, combine the mixed berries, Greek yoghurt, almond milk, protein powder, and honey or maple syrup if using.
2. Blend until smooth and creamy, adding ice cubes if you prefer a colder smoothie.
3. Taste the smoothie and adjust sweetness or consistency by adding more honey/maple syrup or almond milk as needed.
4. Pour the smoothie into a glass and serve immediately.

NUTRITION INFO

Calories: 250 kcal

Protein: 25g

Carbohydrates: 30g

Fat: 3g

Fiber: 5g

Sugar: 20g

Cucumber and Lemon Infused Water

★★★★★

 4 servings    5 minutes

INGREDIENTS

1 medium cucumber, thinly sliced

1 lemon, thinly sliced

8 cups (about 2 liters) of water

Ice cubes (optional)

Fresh mint leaves (optional, for garnish)

DIRECTIONS

1. Wash the cucumber and lemon thoroughly under cold water.
2. Slice the cucumber and lemon into thin rounds.
3. In a large pitcher, add the cucumber and lemon slices.
4. Pour the water into the pitcher, covering the cucumber and lemon slices.
5. Stir gently to combine.
6. Refrigerate for at least 1 hour to allow the flavors to infuse.
7. Serve the infused water over ice cubes, if desired.
8. Garnish with fresh mint leaves for extra freshness.

NUTRITION INFO

Calories: 0
Total Fat: 0g
Cholesterol: 0mg
Sodium: 0mg
Total   Carbohydrates: 0g
Dietary Fiber: 0g
Sugars: 0g
Protein: 0g

Golden Milk Turmeric Latte

 1 servings 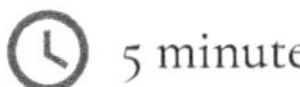 5 minutes

INGREDIENTS

1 cup unsweetened almond milk (or milk of your choice)

1 teaspoon ground turmeric

1/2 teaspoon ground cinnamon

1/4 teaspoon ground ginger

1/8 teaspoon ground black pepper

1 teaspoon honey or maple syrup (optional, for sweetness)

A dash of vanilla extract (optional)

DIRECTIONS

1. In a small saucepan, heat the almond milk over medium heat until it begins to simmer.
2. Whisk in the ground turmeric, cinnamon, ginger, black pepper, and honey or maple syrup if using.
3. Continue to whisk gently until the mixture is well combined and heated through, about 3-4 minutes. Be careful not to boil the mixture.
4. Remove from heat and stir in the vanilla extract if desired.
5. Pour the golden milk turmeric latte into a mug and serve hot.

NUTRITION INFO

Calories: 70 kcal

Total Fat: 2g

Saturated Fat: 0g

Cholesterol: 0mg

Sodium: 170mg

Total Carbohydrates: 12g

Dietary Fiber: 2g

Sugars: 8g

Protein: 1g

Chapter 8

Low Sodium Recipes

Baked Macaroni and Cheese with Broccoli

 6 servings    45 minutes

INGREDIENTS

8 ounces (about 2 cups) elbow macaroni

2 cups broccoli florets, steamed

2 tablespoons unsalted butter

2 tablespoons all-purpose flour

2 cups whole milk

2 cups shredded sharp cheddar cheese

1/2 teaspoon salt

1/4 teaspoon black pepper

1/4 teaspoon paprika (optional)

1/4 cup breadcrumbs (optional)

Cooking spray or butter for greasing the baking dish

NUTRITION INFO

Calories: 395 kcal
Total Fat: 19g
Saturated Fat: 12g
Trans Fat: 0g
Cholesterol: 58mg
Sodium: 542mg
Total Carbohydrates: 36g
Dietary Fiber: 2g
Sugars: 5g
Protein: 20g

DIRECTIONS

1. Preheat your oven to 375°F (190°C). Grease a 9x13-inch baking dish with cooking spray or butter and set aside.
2. Cook the elbow macaroni according to the package instructions until al dente. Drain and set aside.
3. In a large saucepan, melt the butter over medium heat. Once melted, whisk in the flour to form a roux. Cook for 1-2 minutes, stirring constantly, until the roux is golden brown.
4. Gradually pour in the milk, whisking constantly to prevent lumps from forming. Cook for 5-7 minutes, or until the mixture thickens, stirring frequently.
5. Remove the saucepan from the heat and stir in 1 1/2 cups of shredded cheddar cheese until melted and smooth. Season with salt, black pepper, and paprika, if using.
6. Add the cooked macaroni and steamed broccoli to the cheese sauce, stirring until well combined.
7. Transfer the macaroni and cheese mixture to the prepared baking dish, spreading it out evenly.
8. Sprinkle the remaining 1/2 cup of shredded cheddar cheese over the top of the macaroni mixture. If desired, sprinkle breadcrumbs evenly over the cheese layer.
9. Bake in the preheated oven for 20-25 minutes, or until the cheese is bubbly and golden brown on top.
10. Remove from the oven and let it cool for a few minutes before serving. Enjoy hot!

Lemon Herb Grilled Chicken Breast

 4 servings  25 minutes

INGREDIENTS

4 boneless, skinless chicken breasts

2 tablespoons olive oil

2 cloves garlic, minced

Zest and juice of 1 lemon

1 teaspoon dried thyme

1 teaspoon dried rosemary

1 teaspoon dried oregano

Salt and pepper to taste

Lemon wedges (for serving)

Fresh chopped parsley (for garnish)

DIRECTIONS

1. In a small bowl, whisk together olive oil, minced garlic, lemon zest, lemon juice, dried thyme, dried rosemary, dried oregano, salt, and pepper.
2. Place the chicken breasts in a shallow dish or a resealable plastic bag. Pour the marinade over the chicken, making sure each piece is well coated. Marinate in the refrigerator for at least 30 minutes, or up to 4 hours for maximum flavor.
3. Preheat the grill to medium-high heat. Remove the chicken breasts from the marinade and discard any excess marinade.
4. Grill the chicken breasts for 6-8 minutes per side, or until they are cooked through and no longer pink in the center. The internal temperature should reach 165°F (75°C).
5. Once cooked, remove the chicken from the grill and let it rest for a few minutes before serving.
6. Serve the lemon herb grilled chicken breasts with lemon wedges on the side for an extra burst of flavor. Garnish with fresh chopped parsley, if desired.
7. Enjoy your flavorful and healthy lemon herb grilled chicken breasts!

NUTRITION INFO

Calories: 200 kcal

Protein: 25g

Carbohydrates: 2g

Fat: 9g

Saturated Fat: 2g

Cholesterol: 75mg

Sodium: 400mg

Fiber: 1g

Sugar: 0g

Roasted Vegetable Medley with Herbs

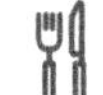 4 servings  40 minutes

INGREDIENTS

2 cups cherry tomatoes, halved

1 medium zucchini, sliced into rounds

1 medium yellow squash, sliced into rounds

1 red bell pepper, sliced into strips

1 yellow bell pepper, sliced into strips

1 red onion, sliced

3 tablespoons olive oil

3 cloves garlic, minced

1 teaspoon dried thyme

1 teaspoon dried rosemary

1 teaspoon dried oregano

Salt and pepper to taste

Fresh herbs (such as parsley or basil) for garnish (optional)

DIRECTIONS

1. Preheat your oven to 425°F (220°C) and line a baking sheet with parchment paper or aluminum foil.
2. In a large mixing bowl, combine the cherry tomatoes, zucchini, yellow squash, bell peppers, and red onion.
3. In a small bowl, whisk together the olive oil, minced garlic, dried thyme, dried rosemary, and dried oregano.
4. Pour the olive oil mixture over the vegetables and toss until evenly coated.
5. Spread the vegetables in a single layer on the prepared baking sheet.
6. Season with salt and pepper to taste.
7. Roast in the preheated oven for 20-25 minutes, or until the vegetables are tender and slightly caramelized, stirring halfway through cooking.
8. Once done, remove from the oven and transfer the roasted vegetable medley to a serving dish.
9. Garnish with fresh herbs if desired.
10. Serve hot as a side dish or over cooked quinoa or brown rice for a wholesome meal.

NUTRITION INFO

Calories: 145 kcal	Total
Total Fat: 9g	Carbohydrates: 15g
Saturated Fat: 1g	Dietary Fiber: 4g
Trans Fat: 0g	Sugars: 7g
Cholesterol: 0mg	Protein: 3g
Sodium: 15mg	

Bean and Vegetable Chili

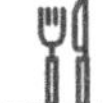 6 servings  55 minutes

INGREDIENTS

1 tablespoon olive oil

1 onion, diced

2 cloves garlic, minced

1 red bell pepper, diced

1 green bell pepper, diced

2 carrots, diced

1 zucchini, diced

1 cup corn kernels (fresh or frozen)

1 can (15 oz) black beans, drained and rinsed

1 can (15 oz) kidney beans, drained and rinsed

1 can (15 oz) diced tomatoes

1 cup vegetable broth

2 tablespoons tomato paste

2 teaspoons chili powder

1 teaspoon cumin

1 teaspoon paprika

Salt and pepper to taste

Optional toppings: chopped fresh cilantro, avocado slices, shredded cheese, sour cream

DIRECTIONS

1. Heat olive oil in a large pot over medium heat. Add diced onion and minced garlic, sauté until softened and fragrant, about 3-4 minutes.

2. Add diced bell peppers, carrots, and zucchini to the pot. Cook for another 5 minutes, stirring occasionally.

3. Stir in corn kernels, black beans, kidney beans, diced tomatoes, vegetable broth, tomato paste, chili powder, cumin, paprika, salt, and pepper.

4. Bring the chili to a simmer, then reduce heat to low. Cover and let it simmer for 30-35 minutes, stirring occasionally.

5. Once the vegetables are tender and the flavors have melded together, taste the chili and adjust seasoning if needed.

6. Serve hot, garnished with chopped fresh cilantro, avocado slices, shredded cheese, or sour cream if desired.

NUTRITION INFO

Calories: 280 kcal

Protein: 12g

Fat: 2g

Carbohydrates: 52g

Fiber: 15g

Sodium: 480mg

Baked Cod with Mediterranean Salsa

 4 servings    20 minutes

INGREDIENTS

4 cod fillets (about 6 ounces each)

2 tablespoons olive oil

1 teaspoon dried oregano

1 teaspoon dried basil

1 teaspoon garlic powder

Salt and pepper to taste

Mediterranean Salsa:

1 cup cherry tomatoes, quartered

1/2 cup diced cucumber

1/4 cup chopped red onion

1/4 cup chopped Kalamata olives

2 tablespoons chopped fresh parsley

2 tablespoons chopped fresh basil

1 tablespoon extra virgin olive oil

1 tablespoon red wine vinegar

DIRECTIONS

1. Preheat your oven to 400°F (200°C). Line a baking sheet with parchment paper or lightly grease it.
2. Place the cod fillets on the prepared baking sheet. Drizzle them with olive oil and sprinkle with dried oregano, basil, garlic powder, salt, and pepper.
3. Bake the cod in the preheated oven for 15-20 minutes, or until it flakes easily with a fork and reaches an internal temperature of 145°F (63°C).
4. While the cod is baking, prepare the Mediterranean salsa. In a bowl, combine the cherry tomatoes, diced cucumber, chopped red onion, Kalamata olives, fresh parsley, and fresh basil.
5. Drizzle the salsa with extra virgin olive oil and red wine vinegar. Season with salt and pepper to taste. Toss gently to combine.
6. Once the cod is cooked, remove it from the oven and serve it topped with the Mediterranean salsa.

NUTRITION INFO

Calories: 285 kcal

Protein: 29g

Fat: 14g

Carbohydrates: 7g

Fiber: 2g

Sugar: 3g

Sodium: 360mg

Quinoa Salad with Lemon Vinaigrette

 4 servings    15 minutes

INGREDIENTS

1 cup quinoa, rinsed

2 cups water

1 cucumber, diced

1 red bell pepper, diced

1/4 cup red onion, finely chopped

1/4 cup fresh parsley, chopped

1/4 cup feta cheese, crumbled (optional)

Salt and pepper to taste

For the Lemon Vinaigrette:

1/4 cup extra virgin olive oil

Juice of 1 lemon

1 teaspoon honey or maple syrup (optional)

1 teaspoon Dijon mustard

1 clove garlic, minced

DIRECTIONS

1. In a medium saucepan, bring the water to a boil. Add the rinsed quinoa and reduce heat to low. Cover and simmer for about 15 minutes, or until quinoa is cooked and water is absorbed. Remove from heat and let it cool.
2. In a small bowl, whisk together the ingredients for the lemon vinaigrette: olive oil, lemon juice, honey or maple syrup (if using), Dijon mustard, minced garlic, salt, and pepper. Set aside.
3. In a large mixing bowl, combine the cooked quinoa, diced cucumber, diced red bell pepper, chopped red onion, and chopped parsley. Toss to combine.
4. Pour the prepared lemon vinaigrette over the quinoa salad and toss until everything is evenly coated.
5. If desired, sprinkle crumbled feta cheese over the salad before serving.
6. Season with additional salt and pepper to taste, if needed.
7. Serve immediately, or refrigerate for at least 30 minutes to allow the flavors to meld before serving.

NUTRITION INFO

Calories: 290 kcal	Total
Total Fat: 16g	Carbohydrates: 31g
Saturated Fat: 3g	Dietary Fiber: 4g
Cholesterol: 6mg	Sugars: 4g
Sodium: 146mg	Protein: 7g

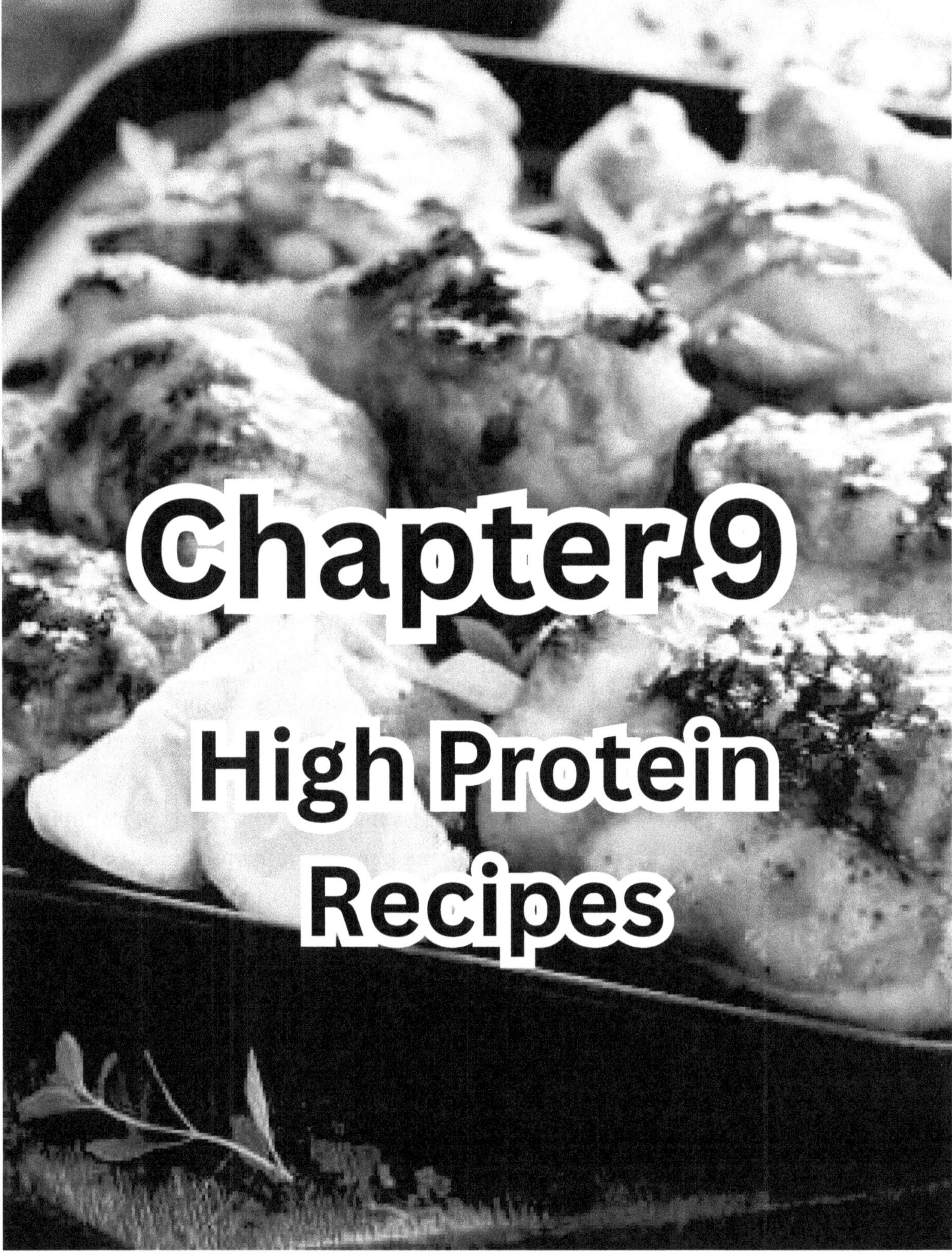
Chapter 9
High Protein
Recipes

Turkey and Quinoa Stuffed Bell Peppers

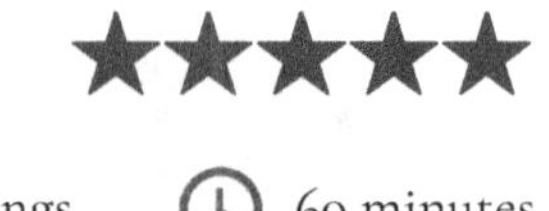

★★★★★

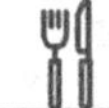 4 servings　 60 minutes

INGREDIENTS

4 large bell peppers (any color), halved and seeds removed

1 cup quinoa, rinsed

1 lb ground turkey

1 small onion, finely chopped

2 cloves garlic, minced

1 can (14.5 oz) diced tomatoes, drained

1 cup spinach, chopped

1 teaspoon dried oregano

1 teaspoon dried basil

Salt and pepper, to taste

1 cup shredded mozzarella cheese (optional)

Fresh parsley, chopped (for garnish)

NUTRITION INFO

Calories: 385 kcal	Total
Total Fat: 12g	Carbohydrates: 35g
Saturated Fat: 4g	Dietary Fiber: 6g
Cholesterol: 81mg	Sugars: 7g
Sodium: 314mg	Protein: 33g

DIRECTIONS

1. Preheat your oven to 375°F (190°C).
2. In a medium saucepan, bring 2 cups of water to a boil. Add the quinoa, reduce heat to low, cover, and simmer for about 15 minutes or until the quinoa is cooked and the water is absorbed.
3. While the quinoa is cooking, heat a large skillet over medium heat. Add the ground turkey and cook until browned, breaking it up with a spoon as it cooks.
4. Add the chopped onion and garlic to the skillet with the turkey, and cook for another 2-3 minutes until the onion is softened.
5. Stir in the diced tomatoes, chopped spinach, dried oregano, dried basil, cooked quinoa, salt, and pepper. Cook for an additional 2-3 minutes until everything is heated through and well combined.
6. Arrange the halved bell peppers in a baking dish, cut side up. Spoon the turkey and quinoa mixture evenly into each pepper half.
7. If desired, sprinkle shredded mozzarella cheese on top of each stuffed pepper.
8. Cover the baking dish with foil and bake in the preheated oven for 25-30 minutes, or until the peppers are tender.
9. Remove the foil and bake for an additional 5-10 minutes, or until the cheese is melted and bubbly.
10. Garnish with chopped fresh parsley before serving.

Chickpea and Spinach Curry

 4 servings    35 minutes

INGREDIENTS

2 tablespoons olive oil

1 onion, finely chopped

3 cloves garlic, minced

1 tablespoon fresh ginger, grated

1 teaspoon ground cumin

1 teaspoon ground coriander

1 teaspoon turmeric

1/2 teaspoon paprika

1/4 teaspoon cayenne pepper (optional, adjust to taste)

1 can (15 ounces) chickpeas, drained and rinsed

1 can (14 ounces) diced tomatoes

1 can (14 ounces) coconut milk

4 cups fresh spinach leaves

Salt and pepper, to taste

Fresh cilantro, chopped (for garnish)

DIRECTIONS

1. Heat the olive oil in a large skillet or pot over medium heat. Add the chopped onion and cook until softened, about 5 minutes.
2. Add the minced garlic and grated ginger to the skillet, and cook for an additional 1–2 minutes until fragrant.
3. Stir in the ground cumin, ground coriander, turmeric, paprika, and cayenne pepper (if using). Cook for another minute to toast the spices.
4. Add the drained chickpeas, diced tomatoes (with their juices), and coconut milk to the skillet. Stir well to combine.
5. Bring the curry to a simmer and let it cook for 15 minutes, stirring occasionally, until the sauce has thickened slightly.
6. Add the fresh spinach leaves to the skillet and stir until wilted.
7. Season the curry with salt and pepper to taste. Adjust the seasoning as needed.
8. Serve the chickpea and spinach curry hot, garnished with fresh cilantro. Enjoy with cooked rice or naan bread.

NUTRITION INFO

Calories: 380 kcal

Protein: 10g

Fat: 25g

Carbohydrates: 30g

Fiber: 8g

Sugar: 7g

Sodium: 650mg

Grilled Steak Salad with Balsamic Glaze

 4 servings  30 minutes

INGREDIENTS

1 lb (450g) sirloin steak

6 cups mixed salad greens (such as baby spinach, arugula, and romaine)

1 cup cherry tomatoes, halved

1/2 red onion, thinly sliced

1/4 cup crumbled feta cheese

Salt and pepper to taste

Olive oil for grilling

For the Balsamic Glaze:

1/2 cup balsamic vinegar

2 tablespoons honey

1 clove garlic, minced

DIRECTIONS

1. Preheat grill to medium-high heat.
2. Season the steak generously with salt and pepper on both sides.
3. Grill the steak for about 4-5 minutes per side for medium-rare, or adjust cooking time according to desired doneness. Remove from grill and let it rest for 5 minutes before slicing.
4. While the steak is resting, prepare the balsamic glaze. In a small saucepan, combine balsamic vinegar, honey, minced garlic, salt, and pepper. Bring to a simmer over medium heat and cook until the glaze is slightly thickened, about 5-7 minutes. Remove from heat and set aside.
5. In a large bowl, toss together the mixed salad greens, cherry tomatoes, and red onion slices.
6. Slice the grilled steak thinly against the grain.
7. Arrange the salad on serving plates, top with sliced steak, and drizzle with balsamic glaze.
8. Sprinkle crumbled feta cheese over the top and serve immediately.

NUTRITION INFO

Calories: 320 kcal

Protein: 26g

Carbohydrates: 14g

Fat: 17g

Fiber: 3g

Sugar: 9g

Sodium: 380mg

Tofu and Vegetable Stir-Fry

 4 servings  30 minutes

INGREDIENTS

1 block (14 oz) extra-firm tofu, pressed and cubed

2 tablespoons soy sauce (or tamari for gluten-free option)

2 tablespoons hoisin sauce

1 tablespoon rice vinegar

1 tablespoon sesame oil

2 cloves garlic, minced

1 teaspoon fresh ginger, grated

2 cups mixed vegetables (such as bell peppers, broccoli, snap peas, carrots), sliced

2 green onions, chopped

2 tablespoons vegetable oil, for cooking

DIRECTIONS

1. In a small bowl, whisk together soy sauce, hoisin sauce, rice vinegar, sesame oil, minced garlic, and grated ginger to make the sauce. Set aside.
2. Heat vegetable oil in a large skillet or wok over medium-high heat.
3. Add cubed tofu to the skillet and cook until golden brown on all sides, about 5-7 minutes. Remove tofu from the skillet and set aside.
4. In the same skillet, add a bit more oil if needed, then add mixed vegetables. Stir-fry for 5-7 minutes or until vegetables are tender-crisp.
5. Return the cooked tofu to the skillet with the vegetables.
6. Pour the sauce over the tofu and vegetables. Stir well to combine and coat everything evenly. Cook for an additional 2-3 minutes until heated through.
7. Sprinkle chopped green onions over the stir-fry and remove from heat.
8. Serve hot with cooked rice or noodles.

NUTRITION INFO

Calories: 240 kcal Fat: 14g

Protein: 12g Saturated Fat: 2g

Carbohydrates: 18g Cholesterol: 0mg

Fiber: 4g Sodium: 630mg

Sugars: 6g

Greek Yogurt Chicken Skewers with Tzatziki Sauce

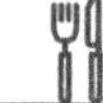 4 servings  30 minutes

INGREDIENTS

1 lb (450g) boneless, skinless chicken breasts, cut into bite-sized pieces

1 cup Greek yogurt

2 tablespoons olive oil

2 cloves garlic, minced

1 teaspoon dried oregano

1 teaspoon dried thyme

1 teaspoon paprika

Salt and pepper to taste

Wooden skewers, soaked in water for 30 minutes

For the Tzatziki Sauce:

1 cup Greek yogurt

1/2 cucumber, grated and squeezed to remove excess moisture

1 clove garlic, minced

1 tablespoon lemon juice

1 tablespoon chopped fresh dill (or 1 teaspoon dried dill)

DIRECTIONS

1. In a mixing bowl, combine the Greek yoghurt, olive oil, minced garlic, dried oregano, dried thyme, paprika, salt, and pepper. Stir until well combined.

2. Add the chicken pieces to the yoghurt marinade, making sure each piece is well coated. Cover and refrigerate for at least 1 hour, or overnight for the best flavour.

3. While the chicken is marinating, prepare the tzatziki sauce. In another bowl, combine the Greek yoghurt, grated cucumber, minced garlic, lemon juice, chopped dill, salt, and pepper. Mix well and refrigerate until ready to serve.

4. Preheat the grill or grill pan over medium-high heat. Thread the marinated chicken pieces onto the soaked wooden skewers.

5. Grill the chicken skewers for about 4-5 minutes on each side, or until cooked through and slightly charred.

6. Serve the grilled chicken skewers with the tzatziki sauce on the side for dipping.

NUTRITION INFO

Calories: 280

Total Fat: 11g

Saturated Fat: 2g

Cholesterol: 85mg

Sodium: 170mg

Total Carbohydrate: 7g

Dietary Fiber: 1g

Sugars: 4g

Protein: 35g

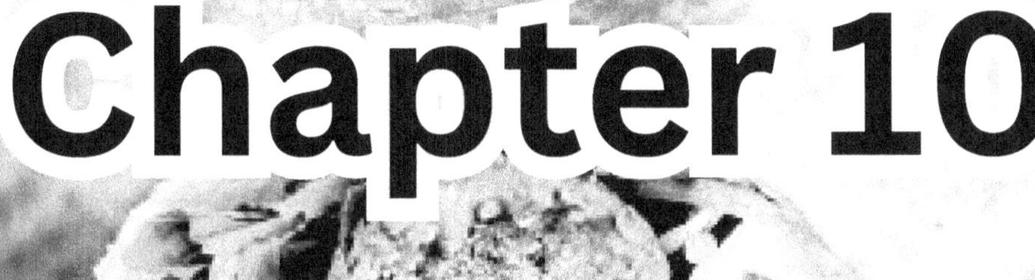
Chapter 10
Gluten-Free
Recipes

Cauliflower Crust Pizza with Vegetables

 4 servings   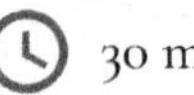 30 minutes

INGREDIENTS

1 medium head of cauliflower, grated (about 3 cups)

1/2 cup shredded mozzarella cheese

1/4 cup grated Parmesan cheese

1 large egg, lightly beaten

1 teaspoon dried oregano

1/2 teaspoon garlic powder

Salt and black pepper to taste

1/2 cup pizza sauce

1 cup sliced bell peppers (red, green, yellow)

1/2 cup sliced red onion

1/2 cup sliced mushrooms

1/4 cup sliced black olives

1/2 cup shredded mozzarella cheese (for topping)

Fresh basil leaves for garnish (optional)

DIRECTIONS

1. Preheat your oven to 425°F (220°C). Line a baking sheet with parchment paper.
2. Place the grated cauliflower in a microwave-safe bowl and microwave on high for 5-6 minutes, or until softened. Allow it to cool slightly.
3. Once cooled, transfer the cauliflower to a clean kitchen towel or cheesecloth. Squeeze out as much moisture as possible. This step is crucial to ensure a crispy crust.
4. In a mixing bowl, combine the squeezed cauliflower, shredded mozzarella, grated Parmesan, beaten egg, dried oregano, garlic powder, salt, and pepper. Mix until well combined and forms a dough-like consistency.
5. Transfer the cauliflower mixture onto the prepared baking sheet. Using your hands, press and shape the mixture into a round pizza crust, about 1/4 inch thick.
6. Bake the cauliflower crust in the preheated oven for 15-20 minutes, or until golden brown and firm.
7. Once the crust is baked, remove it from the oven and spread the pizza sauce evenly over the crust, leaving a small border around the edges.
8. Arrange the sliced bell peppers, red onion, mushrooms, and black olives over the pizza sauce. Sprinkle the remaining shredded mozzarella cheese on top.
9. Return the pizza to the oven and bake for an additional 10-12 minutes, or until the cheese is melted and bubbly.
10. Once done, remove the pizza from the oven and let it cool for a few minutes. Garnish with fresh basil leaves if desired.
11. Slice the cauliflower crust pizza into wedges and serve hot. Enjoy your delicious and nutritious vegetable-packed pizza!

NUTRITION INFO

Calories: 220	Total
Total Fat: 10g	Carbohydrates: 22g
Saturated Fat: 4g	Dietary Fiber: 7g
Cholesterol: 20mg	Sugars: 5g
Sodium: 540mg	Protein: 15g

Gluten-Free Pasta Primavera

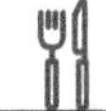 4 servings  30 minutes

INGREDIENTS

8 oz gluten-free pasta (such as brown rice or quinoa pasta)
2 tablespoons olive oil
2 cloves garlic, minced
1 small red onion, thinly sliced
1 cup cherry tomatoes, halved
1 small zucchini, thinly sliced
1 small yellow squash, thinly sliced
1 cup broccoli florets
1 cup sliced bell peppers (any color)
1 cup baby spinach leaves
1/4 cup fresh basil leaves, chopped
Salt and pepper to taste
1/4 cup grated Parmesan cheese (optional, omit for dairy-free or vegan)

DIRECTIONS

1. Cook the gluten-free pasta according to the package instructions until al dente. Drain and set aside.
2. In a large skillet, heat the olive oil over medium heat. Add the minced garlic and sliced red onion, and sauté until softened, about 2-3 minutes.
3. Add the cherry tomatoes, zucchini, yellow squash, broccoli, and bell peppers to the skillet. Cook, stirring occasionally, until the vegetables are tender but still crisp, about 5-7 minutes.
4. Add the cooked pasta and baby spinach to the skillet. Stir well to combine and cook for an additional 2-3 minutes until the spinach is wilted.
5. Season the pasta primavera with salt and pepper to taste. Stir in the chopped basil leaves.
6. Serve the gluten-free pasta primavera hot, topped with grated Parmesan cheese if desired.

NUTRITION INFO

Calories: 320	Total
Total Fat: 12g	Carbohydrates: 48g
Saturated Fat: 2g	Dietary Fiber: 8g
Cholesterol: 0mg	Sugars: 6g
Sodium: 450mg	Protein: 10g

Coconut Flour Banana Pancakes

 8 servings 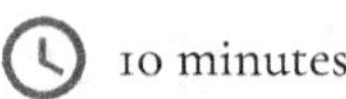 10 minutes

INGREDIENTS

2 ripe bananas, mashed

4 eggs

1/4 cup coconut flour

1/2 teaspoon baking powder

1/2 teaspoon vanilla extract

Pinch of salt

Coconut oil, for cooking

DIRECTIONS

1. In a mixing bowl, combine mashed bananas, eggs, coconut flour, baking powder, vanilla extract, and salt. Mix well until smooth batter forms.
2. Heat a non-stick skillet or griddle over medium heat and lightly grease with coconut oil.
3. Pour about 1/4 cup of batter onto the skillet for each pancake. Cook until bubbles form on the surface, then flip and cook until golden brown on the other side.
4. Repeat with the remaining batter.
5. Serve warm with your favorite toppings such as fresh fruit, Greek yogurt, or maple syrup.

NUTRITION INFO

Calories: 82 kcal	Total
Total Fat: 3.5 g	Carbohydrates: 9 g
Saturated Fat: 2 g	Dietary Fiber: 2 g
Cholesterol: 93 mg	Sugars: 4 g
Sodium: 90 mg	Protein: 4 g

Zucchini Noodles with Pesto and Cherry Tomatoes

 4 servings 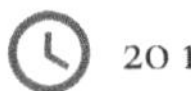 20 minutes

INGREDIENTS

4 medium zucchini, spiralized into noodles
1 cup cherry tomatoes, halved
1/4 cup pine nuts, toasted
1/2 cup fresh basil leaves
2 cloves garlic
1/4 cup grated Parmesan cheese (optional, omit for dairy-free version)
1/4 cup extra virgin olive oil
Salt and pepper to taste
Red pepper flakes (optional, for added heat)

DIRECTIONS

1. In a food processor, combine the basil, garlic, pine nuts, and Parmesan cheese (if using). Pulse until finely chopped.
2. With the food processor running, slowly pour in the olive oil until the mixture is smooth and well combined. Season with salt and pepper to taste. If desired, add red pepper flakes for some heat.
3. In a large skillet, heat a drizzle of olive oil over medium heat. Add the cherry tomatoes and cook for 2-3 minutes until they start to soften.
4. Add the zucchini noodles to the skillet and toss with the cherry tomatoes until heated through, about 2-3 minutes.
5. Remove the skillet from heat and add the pesto sauce to the zucchini noodles. Toss until the noodles are evenly coated with the pesto.
6. Serve the zucchini noodles with additional grated Parmesan cheese and a sprinkle of toasted pine nuts, if desired. Enjoy

NUTRITION INFO

Calories: 230	Total
Total Fat: 20g	Carbohydrates: 8g
Saturated Fat: 3g	Dietary Fiber: 3g
Cholesterol: 0mg	Sugars: 5g
Sodium: 120mg	Protein: 5g

Almond Flour Blueberry Muffins

 12 servings  40 minutes

INGREDIENTS

2 cups almond flour

1/4 cup coconut flour

1/2 teaspoon baking soda

1/4 teaspoon salt

3 large eggs

1/4 cup honey or maple syrup

1/4 cup coconut oil, melted

1 teaspoon vanilla extract

1 cup fresh blueberries

DIRECTIONS

1. Preheat your oven to 350°F (175°C). Line a muffin tin with paper liners or grease well.
2. In a large bowl, whisk together the almond flour, coconut flour, baking soda, and salt until well combined.
3. In another bowl, beat the eggs, then add the honey or maple syrup, melted coconut oil, and vanilla extract. Mix until smooth.
4. Pour the wet ingredients into the dry ingredients and stir until just combined. Be careful not to overmix.
5. Gently fold in the blueberries until evenly distributed throughout the batter.
6. Spoon the batter into the prepared muffin tin, filling each cup about 2/3 full.
7. Bake in the preheated oven for 20-25 minutes, or until the muffins are golden brown and a toothpick inserted into the center comes out clean.
8. Remove from the oven and allow the muffins to cool in the pan for 5 minutes before transferring them to a wire rack to cool completely.

NUTRITION INFO

Calories: 180 kcal

Total Fat: 13g

Saturated Fat: 4g

Trans Fat: 0g

Cholesterol: 47mg

Sodium: 117mg

Total Carbohydrates: 13g

Dietary Fiber: 2g

Sugars: 8g

Protein: 5g

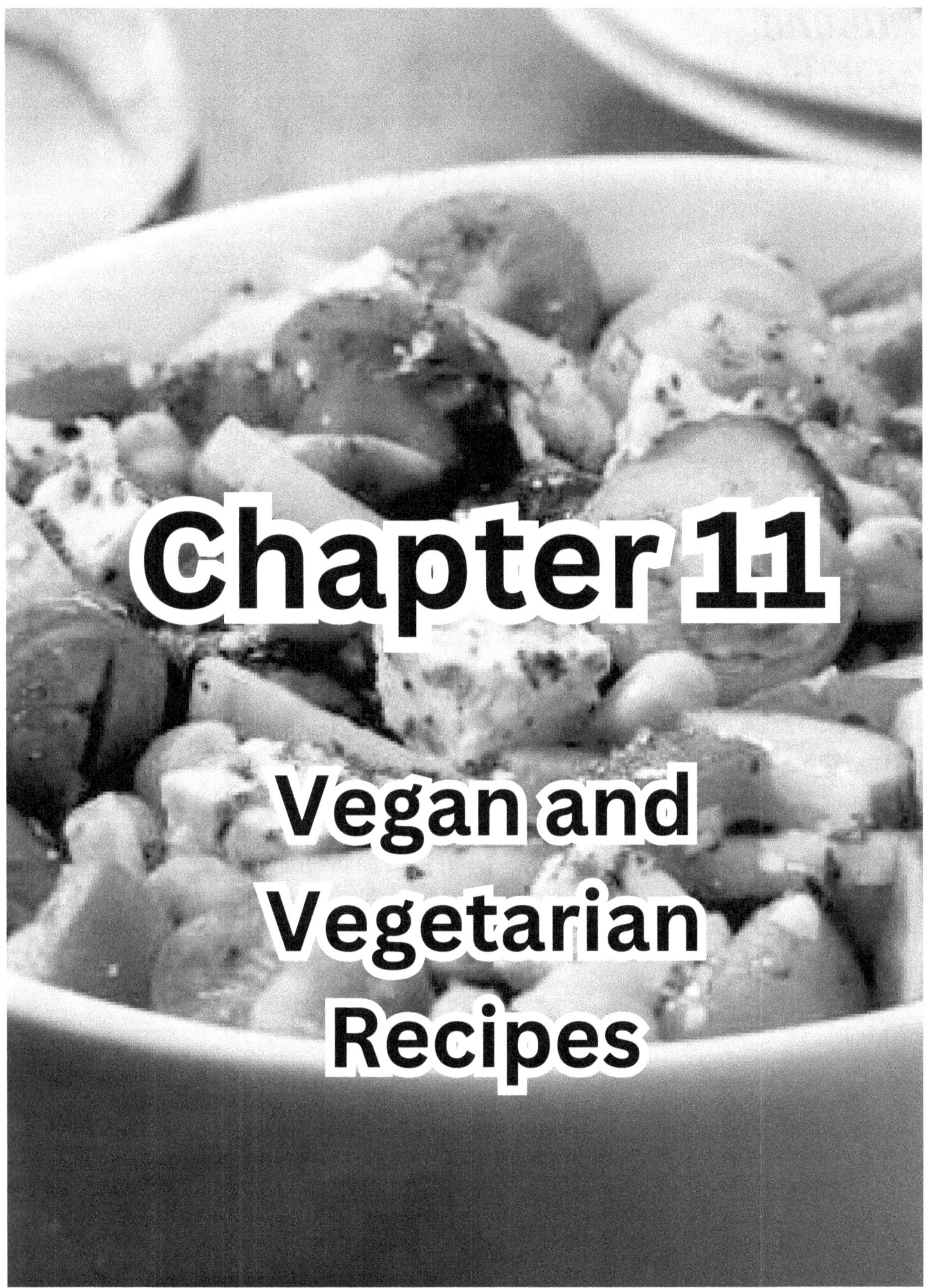

Chapter 11
Vegan and Vegetarian Recipes

Lentil and Vegetable Shepherd's Pie

 6 servings  1 hour 15 minutes

INGREDIENTS

2 lbs (about 1 kg) potatoes, peeled and chopped

1/2 cup unsweetened almond milk (or any milk of your choice)

2 tablespoons vegan butter or olive oil

Salt and pepper to taste

For the lentil and vegetable filling:

1 cup green or brown lentils, rinsed and drained

2 cups vegetable broth

1 tablespoon olive oil

1 onion, diced

2 carrots, diced

2 celery stalks, diced

2 cloves garlic, minced

1 teaspoon dried thyme

1 teaspoon dried rosemary

1 teaspoon paprika

Salt and pepper to taste

1 cup frozen peas

1 cup frozen corn

2 tablespoons tomato paste

1 tablespoon soy sauce or tamari

2 tablespoons all-purpose flour (or gluten-free flour)

NUTRITION INFO

Calories: 320 kcal

Protein: 12g

Fat: 8g

Carbohydrates: 52g

Fiber: 10g

Sugar: 10g

Sodium: 550mg

DIRECTIONS

1. Preheat your oven to 375°F (190°C).
2. Place the chopped potatoes in a large pot and cover with water. Bring to a boil and cook for about 15-20 minutes, or until the potatoes are fork-tender.
3. While the potatoes are cooking, prepare the lentil and vegetable filling. In a separate pot, combine the lentils and vegetable broth. Bring to a boil, then reduce the heat and simmer for about 15-20 minutes, or until the lentils are tender but not mushy. Drain any excess liquid and set aside.
4. In a large skillet, heat the olive oil over medium heat. Add the diced onion, carrots, and celery, and cook for about 5-7 minutes, or until softened. Add the minced garlic, dried thyme, dried rosemary, paprika, salt, and pepper, and cook for an additional 2 minutes.
5. Stir in the frozen peas and corn, tomato paste, and soy sauce. Sprinkle the flour over the mixture and stir until well combined. Cook for another 2-3 minutes.
6. Add the cooked lentils to the skillet and stir until everything is evenly mixed. Remove from heat and transfer the lentil and vegetable mixture to a large baking dish.
7. Once the potatoes are cooked, drain them and return them to the pot. Add the almond milk and vegan butter (or olive oil) to the pot with the potatoes. Mash until smooth and creamy. Season with salt and pepper to taste.
8. Spread the mashed potatoes evenly over the lentil and vegetable filling in the baking dish.
9. Place the baking dish in the preheated oven and bake for about 25-30 minutes, or until the mashed potatoes are lightly golden on top.
10. Remove from the oven and let cool for a few minutes before serving. Enjoy your delicious Lentil and Vegetable Shepherd's Pie!

Vegan Buddha Bowl
with Quinoa and Roasted Vegetables

★★★★★

 4 serving   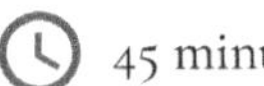 45 minutes

INGREDIENTS

1 cup quinoa, rinsed

2 cups water or vegetable broth

1 medium sweet potato, peeled and diced

2 cups broccoli florets

1 medium red bell pepper, sliced

1 medium zucchini, sliced

1 tablespoon olive oil

1 teaspoon garlic powder

1 teaspoon smoked paprika

Salt and pepper to taste

1 avocado, sliced

1 cup cherry tomatoes, halved

4 tablespoons tahini dressing (store-bought or homemade)

DIRECTIONS

1. Preheat your oven to 400°F (200°C).
2. In a saucepan, bring the water or vegetable broth to a boil. Add the quinoa, reduce the heat to low, cover, and simmer for 15-20 minutes, or until the quinoa is cooked and the liquid is absorbed. Fluff with a fork and set aside.
3. Meanwhile, spread the diced sweet potato, broccoli florets, sliced red bell pepper, and sliced zucchini on a baking sheet. Drizzle with olive oil and sprinkle with garlic powder, smoked paprika, salt, and pepper. Toss to coat evenly.
4. Roast the vegetables in the preheated oven for 20-25 minutes, or until they are tender and lightly browned, stirring halfway through.
5. To assemble the Buddha bowls, divide the cooked quinoa among four bowls. Top each with an equal portion of the roasted vegetables, avocado slices, and cherry tomatoes.
6. Drizzle each bowl with 1 tablespoon of tahini dressing.
7. Serve immediately and enjoy!

NUTRITION INFO

Calories: 380 kcal	Total Carbohydrates: 51g
Total Fat: 17g	
Saturated Fat: 2g	
Trans Fat: 0g	Dietary Fiber: 12g
Cholesterol: 0mg	
Sodium: 70mg	Sugars: 6g
	Protein: 11g

Spinach and Mushroom Stuffed Portobello Mushrooms

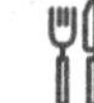 4 serving 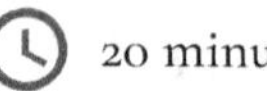 20 minutes

INGREDIENTS

4 large portobello mushrooms

2 cups fresh spinach, chopped

1 cup mushrooms, finely chopped

1 small onion, finely chopped

2 cloves garlic, minced

1/4 cup grated Parmesan cheese

1/4 cup breadcrumbs (gluten-free if desired)

2 tablespoons olive oil

Salt and pepper to taste

Fresh parsley for garnish (optional)

NUTRITION INFO

Calories: 158 kcal	Total
Total Fat: 9g	Carbohydrates: 14g
Saturated Fat: 2g	Dietary Fiber: 3g
Trans Fat: 0g	Sugars: 3g
Cholesterol: 4mg	Protein: 7g
Sodium: 162mg	

DIRECTIONS

1. Preheat your oven to 375°F (190°C). Line a baking sheet with parchment paper or lightly grease it with olive oil.
2. Clean the portobello mushrooms by gently wiping them with a damp cloth or paper towel to remove any dirt. Remove the stems and carefully scoop out the gills using a spoon. Place the mushrooms on the prepared baking sheet, gill-side up.
3. In a skillet, heat 1 tablespoon of olive oil over medium heat. Add the chopped onion and minced garlic, and sauté until softened about 3-4 minutes.
4. Add the chopped mushrooms to the skillet and cook until they release their moisture and start to brown, about 5-6 minutes.
5. Add the chopped spinach to the skillet and cook until wilted, about 2-3 minutes. Season with salt and pepper to taste.
6. Remove the skillet from heat and stir in the grated Parmesan cheese and breadcrumbs until well combined.
7. Spoon the spinach and mushroom mixture into the hollowed-out portobello mushrooms, dividing it evenly among them. Drizzle the stuffed mushrooms with the remaining olive oil.
8. Bake in the preheated oven for 15-20 minutes, or until the mushrooms are tender and the filling is golden brown on top.
9. Garnish with fresh parsley if desired, and serve hot.

Chickpea and Sweet Potato Curry

 4 servings  30 minutes

INGREDIENTS

2 tablespoons olive oil

1 onion, chopped

2 cloves garlic, minced

1 tablespoon ginger, minced

2 teaspoons curry powder

1 teaspoon ground cumin

1 teaspoon ground coriander

1/2 teaspoon turmeric

1/4 teaspoon cayenne pepper (optional, adjust to taste)

2 medium sweet potatoes, peeled and diced

1 can (15 ounces) chickpeas, drained and rinsed

1 can (14 ounces) diced tomatoes

1 can (13.5 ounces) coconut milk

Salt and pepper to taste

Fresh cilantro leaves, for garnish

Cooked rice or naan bread, for serving

DIRECTIONS

1. Heat the olive oil in a large skillet or pot over medium heat. Add the chopped onion and cook until softened, about 5 minutes.
2. Add the minced garlic and ginger to the skillet and cook for another 2 minutes until fragrant.
3. Stir in the curry powder, ground cumin, ground coriander, turmeric, and cayenne pepper (if using). Cook for 1 minute to toast the spices.
4. Add the diced sweet potatoes to the skillet and cook for 5 minutes, stirring occasionally.
5. Pour in the diced tomatoes (with their juices), chickpeas, and coconut milk. Stir to combine everything.
6. Bring the mixture to a simmer, then reduce the heat to low. Cover and let it simmer gently for about 20 minutes, or until the sweet potatoes are tender.
7. Season with salt and pepper to taste. If the curry is too thick, you can add a splash of water to reach your desired consistency.
8. Serve the chickpea and sweet potato curry hot, garnished with fresh cilantro leaves. Enjoy with cooked rice or naan bread.

NUTRITION INFO

Calories: 360	Total Carbohydrates: 38g
Total Fat: 20g	
Saturated Fat: 12g	
Trans Fat: 0g	Dietary Fiber: 8g
Cholesterol: 0mg	Sugars: 9g
Sodium: 450mg	Protein: 9g

Eggplant and Lentil Moussaka

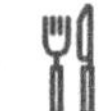 6 servings  60 minutes

INGREDIENTS

2 large eggplants, sliced lengthwise

1 cup dried brown lentils, rinsed and drained

2 cups vegetable broth

1 onion, finely chopped

3 cloves garlic, minced

1 can (14 oz) crushed tomatoes

1 teaspoon dried oregano

1 teaspoon dried basil

Salt and pepper to taste

2 tablespoons olive oil

2 tablespoons all-purpose flour

2 cups milk (dairy or plant-based)

1/4 teaspoon ground nutmeg

1 cup grated Parmesan cheese

NUTRITION INFO

Calories: 320	Total
Total Fat: 12g	Carbohydrates: 42g
Saturated Fat: 4g	Dietary Fiber: 10g
Cholesterol: 20mg	Sugars: 12g
Sodium: 480mg	Protein: 15g

DIRECTIONS

1. Preheat the oven to 375°F (190°C). Grease a 9x13 inch baking dish.
2. Place the sliced eggplants on a baking sheet and brush both sides with olive oil. Bake in the preheated oven for 15-20 minutes, or until tender. Remove from the oven and set aside.
3. In a medium saucepan, combine the lentils and vegetable broth. Bring to a boil, then reduce the heat and simmer for 20-25 minutes, or until the lentils are tender and most of the liquid is absorbed. Remove from heat and set aside.
4. In a separate pan, heat 1 tablespoon of olive oil over medium heat. Add the chopped onion and garlic, and sauté until softened, about 5 minutes. Add the crushed tomatoes, dried oregano, dried basil, salt, and pepper. Cook for another 5 minutes, then remove from heat.
5. In a small saucepan, heat the remaining 1 tablespoon of olive oil over medium heat. Stir in the flour and cook for 1-2 minutes to form a roux. Gradually whisk in the milk until smooth. Cook, stirring constantly, until the sauce thickens, about 5 minutes. Season with nutmeg, salt, and pepper.
6. To assemble the moussaka, spread half of the lentil mixture in the bottom of the prepared baking dish. Top with half of the eggplant slices, then half of the tomato sauce. Repeat the layers with the remaining lentil mixture, eggplant slices, and tomato sauce.
7. Pour the white sauce over the top of the moussaka and spread evenly. Sprinkle the grated Parmesan cheese over the sauce.
8. Bake in the preheated oven for 30-35 minutes, or until the top is golden brown and bubbly. Remove from the oven and let it cool for a few minutes before serving.
9. Serve the moussaka warm, garnished with fresh herbs if desired. Enjoy!

CONCLUSION

In the pages of this cookbook, we've looked at more than simply dishes, but also a route to well-being and vitality. The "Lymphedema Diet" cookbook is more than just a collection of recipes; it demonstrates the power of diet in addressing health issues, encouraging balance, and appreciating the pleasures of nourishment.

As we wrap out this culinary adventure, let us reflect on the lessons learnt and the flavours enjoyed. Each dish is a story of care and intention, made using ingredients picked not just for their taste but also for their medicinal capabilities. Every item, from vivid salads to hearty stews, comforting sweets to energizing beverages, has been deliberately crafted to help patients with lymphedema on their path to wellness.

Beyond the kitchen, this cookbook serves as a reminder of the value of self-care and love. It serves as a reminder that what we put into our bodies has an impact not only on our physical health but also on our whole sense of energy. It's a call to appreciate the richness of whole foods, take each meal carefully, and nourish ourselves with kindness and compassion.

As you leave these pages, may you take with you not only recipes but also a renewed awareness of the remarkable link between food and health. May you continue to discover, experiment, and enjoy the many possibilities that the kitchen provides. And may your path to wellness be led by the simple yet deep insight at the heart of this cookbook: that food is more than simply nourishment; it is also a source of healing, happiness, and love.

VAKARE RIMKUTE

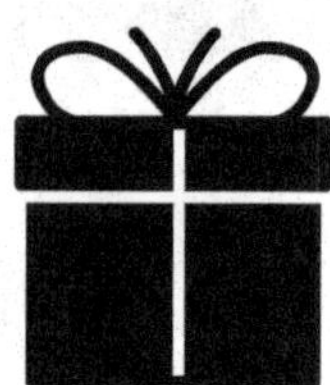

HERE IS YOUR 14 DAYS MEAL PLAN TRACKER WITH A 30-DAY HEALTHY EATING CHALLENGE

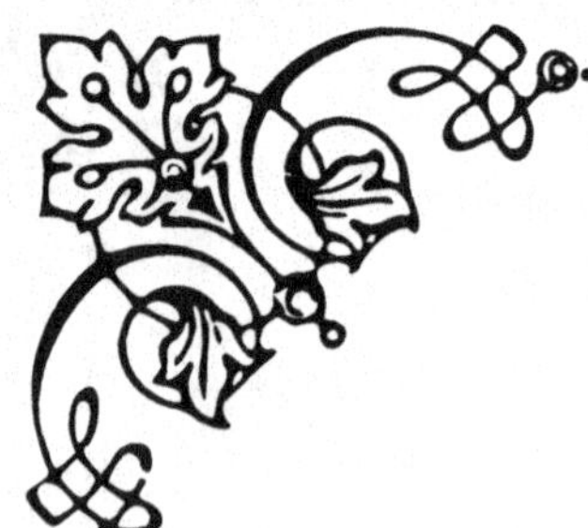

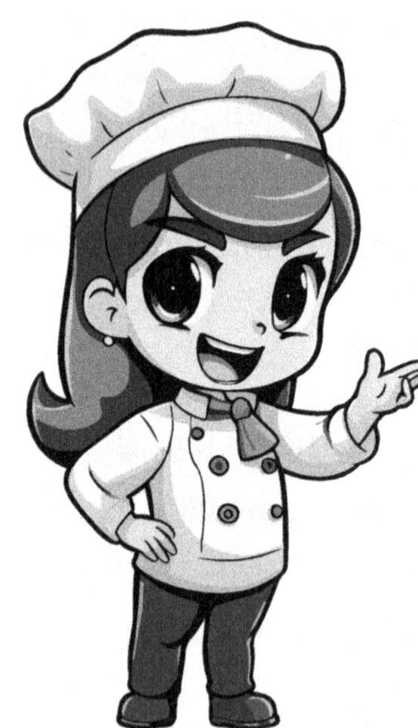

DISCOVER MORE ABOUT MY CULINARY ADVENTURES AND UPCOMING PROJECTS.

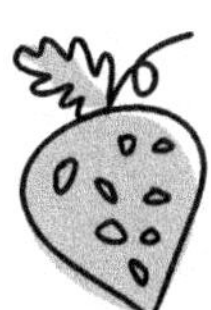

Daily
Meal Planner

	Breakfast:	Lunch:	Dinner:
s			
m			
t			
w			
t			
f			
s			

Daily Meal Planner

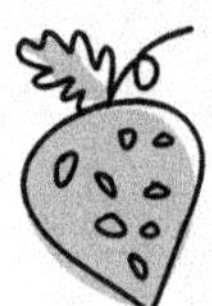

| s | Breakfast: | Lunch: | Dinner: |

| m | Breakfast: | Lunch: | Dinner: |

| t | Breakfast: | Lunch: | Dinner: |

| w | Breakfast: | Lunch: | Dinner: |

| t | Breakfast: | Lunch: | Dinner: |

| f | Breakfast: | Lunch: | Dinner: |

| s | Breakfast: | Lunch: | Dinner: |

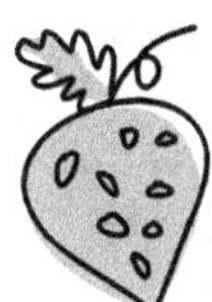

Daily
Meal Planner

| s | Breakfast: | Lunch: | Dinner: |

| m | Breakfast: | Lunch: | Dinner: |

| t | Breakfast: | Lunch: | Dinner: |

| w | Breakfast: | Lunch: | Dinner: |

| t | Breakfast: | Lunch: | Dinner: |

| f | Breakfast: | Lunch: | Dinner: |

| s | Breakfast: | Lunch: | Dinner: |

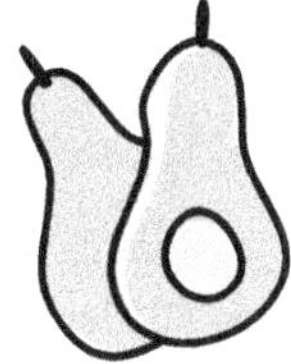

Daily Meal Planner

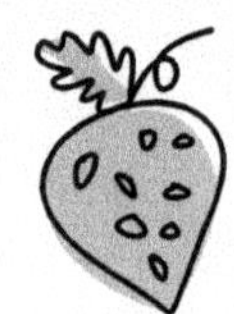

| s | Breakfast: | Lunch: | Dinner: |

| m | Breakfast: | Lunch: | Dinner: |

| t | Breakfast: | Lunch: | Dinner: |

| w | Breakfast: | Lunch: | Dinner: |

| t | Breakfast: | Lunch: | Dinner: |

| f | Breakfast: | Lunch: | Dinner: |

| s | Breakfast: | Lunch: | Dinner: |

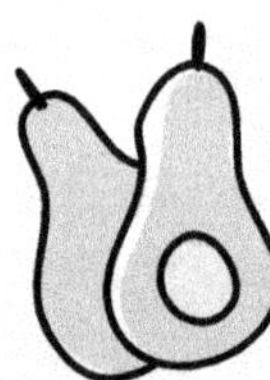

Daily Meal Planner

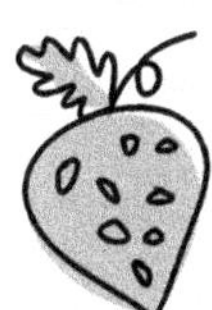

s	Breakfast:	Lunch:	Dinner:
m	Breakfast:	Lunch:	Dinner:
t	Breakfast:	Lunch:	Dinner:
w	Breakfast:	Lunch:	Dinner:
t	Breakfast:	Lunch:	Dinner:
f	Breakfast:	Lunch:	Dinner:
s	Breakfast:	Lunch:	Dinner:

Daily
Meal Planner

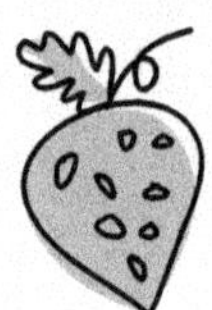

s	Breakfast:	Lunch:	Dinner:
m	Breakfast:	Lunch:	Dinner:
t	Breakfast:	Lunch:	Dinner:
w	Breakfast:	Lunch:	Dinner:
t	Breakfast:	Lunch:	Dinner:
f	Breakfast:	Lunch:	Dinner:
s	Breakfast:	Lunch:	Dinner:

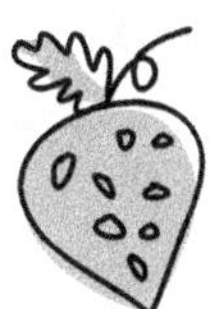

Daily
Meal Planner

| s | Breakfast: | Lunch: | Dinner: |

| m | Breakfast: | Lunch: | Dinner: |

| t | Breakfast: | Lunch: | Dinner: |

| w | Breakfast: | Lunch: | Dinner: |

| t | Breakfast: | Lunch: | Dinner: |

| f | Breakfast: | Lunch: | Dinner: |

| s | Breakfast: | Lunch: | Dinner: |

Daily
Meal Planner

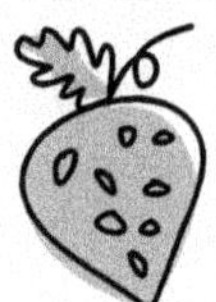

<table>
<tr><td>s</td><td>Breakfast:</td><td>Lunch:</td><td>Dinner:</td></tr>
<tr><td>m</td><td>Breakfast:</td><td>Lunch:</td><td>Dinner:</td></tr>
<tr><td>t</td><td>Breakfast:</td><td>Lunch:</td><td>Dinner:</td></tr>
<tr><td>w</td><td>Breakfast:</td><td>Lunch:</td><td>Dinner:</td></tr>
<tr><td>t</td><td>Breakfast:</td><td>Lunch:</td><td>Dinner:</td></tr>
<tr><td>f</td><td>Breakfast:</td><td>Lunch:</td><td>Dinner:</td></tr>
<tr><td>s</td><td>Breakfast:</td><td>Lunch:</td><td>Dinner:</td></tr>
</table>

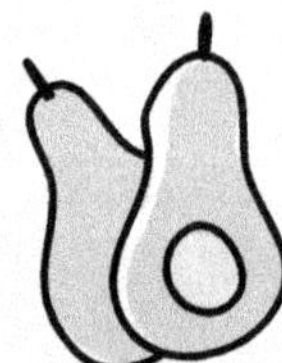

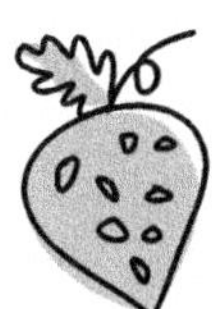

Daily
Meal Planner

| s | Breakfast: | Lunch: | Dinner: |

| m | Breakfast: | Lunch: | Dinner: |

| t | Breakfast: | Lunch: | Dinner: |

| w | Breakfast: | Lunch: | Dinner: |

| t | Breakfast: | Lunch: | Dinner: |

| f | Breakfast: | Lunch: | Dinner: |

| s | Breakfast: | Lunch: | Dinner: |

Daily Meal Planner

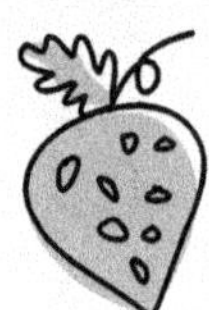

s	Breakfast:	Lunch:	Dinner:
m	Breakfast:	Lunch:	Dinner:
t	Breakfast:	Lunch:	Dinner:
w	Breakfast:	Lunch:	Dinner:
t	Breakfast:	Lunch:	Dinner:
f	Breakfast:	Lunch:	Dinner:
s	Breakfast:	Lunch:	Dinner:

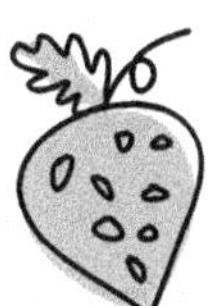

Daily
Meal Planner

s	Breakfast:	Lunch:	Dinner:
m	Breakfast:	Lunch:	Dinner:
t	Breakfast:	Lunch:	Dinner:
w	Breakfast:	Lunch:	Dinner:
t	Breakfast:	Lunch:	Dinner:
f	Breakfast:	Lunch:	Dinner:
s	Breakfast:	Lunch:	Dinner:

Daily Meal Planner

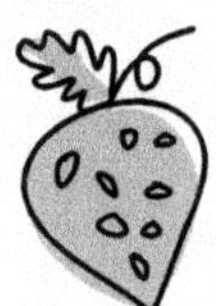

	Breakfast:	Lunch:	Dinner:
s			
m			
t			
w			
t			
f			
s			

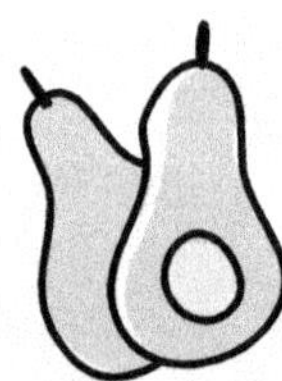

Daily
Meal Planner

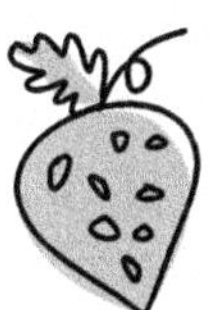

| s | Breakfast: | Lunch: | Dinner: |

| m | Breakfast: | Lunch: | Dinner: |

| t | Breakfast: | Lunch: | Dinner: |

| w | Breakfast: | Lunch: | Dinner: |

| t | Breakfast: | Lunch: | Dinner: |

| f | Breakfast: | Lunch: | Dinner: |

| s | Breakfast: | Lunch: | Dinner: |

Daily
Meal Planner

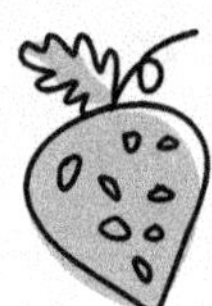

s	Breakfast:	Lunch:	Dinner:
m	Breakfast:	Lunch:	Dinner:
t	Breakfast:	Lunch:	Dinner:
w	Breakfast:	Lunch:	Dinner:
t	Breakfast:	Lunch:	Dinner:
f	Breakfast:	Lunch:	Dinner:
s	Breakfast:	Lunch:	Dinner:

30-Day Healthy Eating Challenge

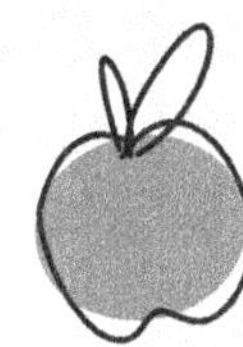

Add some protein	Use whole grains	Fill up on fiber	Don't skip dinner	Try a new veggie
Eat fruits first	Skip dessert	Eliminate sugar	Upgrade your snack	No ice cream
Skip Soda	Mix up your protein	Drink more water	Cut out bad carbs	Eliminate alcohol
Don't skip breakfast	No fast food	Try leafy greens	Morning smoothie	Nutritious breakfast
Eliminate dairy	Avoid salt	Cook at home	Drink herbal tea	Eat vegetables
Snack on fresh fruits	Eliminate coffee	Eat more veggies	Eliminate MSG	Go gluten free

THE AUTHOR

Hello, culinary adventurers!
I'm Vakare Rimkute, a passionate explorer
of the culinary world and a devoted recipe
book writer. With a whisk in one hand and a pen in the other, I traverse
the realms of flavor, seeking to blend tradition with innovation in every
dish I create.

Growing up in the bustling kitchens of my Lithuanian grandmother, I developed an insatiable curiosity for the alchemy of ingredients and the magic they could weave on the palate. From the rustic charm of hearty stews to the delicate intricacies of pastries, my journey through food has been nothing short of a delightful adventure.

After years of experimenting and honing my craft, I found my true calling as a recipe book writer. With each recipe I pen, I aim to capture the essence of culinary culture while infusing it with a touch of modern flair. From comforting classics to bold culinary experiments, my recipes are a reflection of my belief that food should not only nourish the body but also nourish the soul.

So join me on this gastronomic journey, where every page is filled with tantalizing flavors, heartwarming stories, and a dash of humor. Together, let's embark on a culinary adventure that will tickle your taste buds and leave you craving for more. Happy cooking!